C000220363

OVERCOME GASLIGHTING

How To Disarm Manipulative People, Break Free Of
Domestic Violence and Recover From Emotionally Abusive
Relationships

JUNE PRESLEY

Contents

Copyright © 2020 by June Presley- All rights reserved

No part of this publication may be reproduced, stored in a retrieval system or transmitted in any form or by any means, electronic, mechanical, photocopying, recording, scanning or otherwise, except as permitted under Sections 107 or 108 of the 1976 United States Copyright Act, without the prior written permission of the Publisher.

Limit of Liability/Disclaimer of Warranty: The Publisher and the author make no representations or warranties with respect to the accuracy or completeness of the contents of this work and specifically disclaim all warranties, including without limitation warranties of fitness for a particular purpose. No warranty may be created or extended by sales or promotional materials. The advice and strategies contained herein may not be suitable for every situation. This work is sold with the understanding that the Publisher is not engaged in rendering medical, legal, or other professional advice or services. If professional assistance is required, the services of a competent professional person should be sought. Neither the Publisher nor the author shall be liable for damages arising herefrom. The fact that an individual, organization or website is referred to in this work as a citation and/or potential source of further information does not mean that the author or the Publisher endorses the information the individual, organization or website may provide or recommendations they/it may make. Further, readers should be aware that Internet websites listed in this work may have changed or disappeared between when this work was written and when it is read.

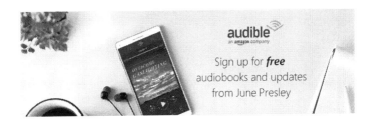

audible
an amazon company

Sign up for *free*
audiobooks and updates
from June Presley

If you want to be the first to receive the audiobook version of this book for free and to get updates and actionable emails from June, then click the image above or the link below.

Go to the URL below to receive free audiobooks and get updates from June.

https://bit.ly/2BAnvfE

Or scan this QR code:

Introduction

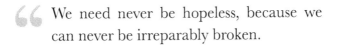

>   We need never be hopeless, because we
>   can never be irreparably broken.

John Green

It can be extremely sad and disturbing when you discover that someone you love has betrayed your trust by deliberately being dishonest and manipulating you. That feeling is like a nightmare that you can't seem to get over. Suddenly, your reality is tipped on its head, and you don't know if you can trust your own memories, let alone the people around you. If you've experienced this scenario at some point in your life, then you already know what I am talking about. If not, you're probably wondering where I am heading with all of this.

The term "gaslighting" comes from the play *Gas*

Light by British dramatist Patrick Hamilton, but it wasn't popularized until the 1944 American film adaptation starring Charles Boyer and Ingrid Bergman. In the film, Boyer plays Gregory, a man conspiring to make his wife Paula (played by Bergman) believe that she has gone mad in order to steal her inheritance. Gregory made Paula believe that she imagined things when she started noticing odd and sneaky behavior on her husband's part. Slowly, the lies and manipulation that Gregory fed his wife begin to manifest in her life as she started to question her sanity. This, in turn, caused other people to begin questioning her sanity as well.

Today, "gaslighting" is a term used to describe behavior and tactics used in emotionally abusive relationships. Unfortunately, this sort of behavior happens all around us. According to Tampa-based psychotherapist Stephanie Sarkis, "Gaslighters are master manipulators, they lie or withhold information, pit people against each other, and always place blame elsewhere, all the while gaining control over those they are gaslighting" (McQuillan 2019).

Initially, gaslighting may begin as what seems like small offenses, like someone telling you that you're overreacting about something. But no matter how little it starts out as—and whichever form of gaslighting it evolves into—you could end up in a cycle where you can't navigate your daily life with a clear, focused, or sound mind. You also won't be able to make decisions for yourself or have a general sense of your own well-being.

This type of psychological abuse goes beyond personal relationships, such as an abusive partner preying on the other, or parents preying on their child. It can also happen in professional relationships, wherein a manipulative boss or co-worker preys on their subordinates or colleagues. In fact, after getting to know about gaslighting in more detail by reading this book, you'll see that gaslighting is all around us. But once you recognize it for what it is, it can do you no harm.

No matter where gaslighting takes place—whether in your personal relationships, at work, between a leader and followers, or anywhere else—it is essential that you understand the red flags associated with gaslighting to avoid becoming a victim. This is the first step to take when finding an escape from an abusive situation.

When you are being gaslighted, the abuser will find a way to make you feel as if you are crazy by constantly making you question your reality. This works because the gaslighter usually knows how to make themselves appear friendly, loving, and empathetic when they need to be. As a victim, it will be hard for you to believe that the person who loves and cares for you so much would ever attempt to hurt you systematically and/or purposefully.

It is important to note that not all differences or

disagreements in perception are a result of gaslighting. Your memories can be unreliable at times because they can be influenced by current assumptions or issues, miscommunication, and faulty information. This is why eye-witness accounts of the same event told by different people can be contradictory. When your relationship has moments where your partner's memory of an event is at odds with yours, do not automatically assume it is gaslighting. That being said, it is always important to be sure of what you are experiencing.

If you have experienced any form of gaslighting, you know how emotionally taxing it can be. The gaslighter will lie and manipulate you in a way that will cause you to start doubting your reality and sanity. Gaslighters will use tactics like blatant lying, turning other people against you, and condemning you for criticizing their behavior. Gaslighting is a harmful form of abuse fueled by uncertainty. If you experience this, you can grow to distrust everything you feel, remember, and hear. One of the most important things you can get as a survivor is validation. What you are feeling and experiencing is real, and you deserve that to be true.

You can benefit from reforming the relationships you pulled back from when you were being abused. Getting sympathy from people can reduce the feeling of shame you feel, and other people can validate your uncertain memories. As you start rebuilding your social circle, you can relearn how to trust yourself and the people around you.

Survivors of gaslighting may wish to seek therapy during their recovery process. A therapist is usually a neutral party that can help you reinforce your sense of reality that got tampered with as a result of your abusive relationship. Therapy can help you to restore your self-esteem and regain control of your life. In some cases, a victim of gaslighting may develop mental health issues, such as Post Traumatic Stress Disorder (PTSD), depression, or severe anxiety. A therapist can also help with this by providing support and necessary reinforcement. With time, you will be able to recover.

We all can be jerks every now and then, but there are a selected few that have adopted this behavior as a lifetime career and use it to undermine you. Whether it is a jealous friend, a vindictive coworker, or a controlling boss that's giving you constant emotional abuse, it is time to put a stop to it.

As a professional that specializes in victims of emotional abuse, I have seen a lot of people through leaving an abusive relationship; and I can safely say that I know how challenging the recovery process is. After seeing case after case of a partner denying the words and experiences of the other, I sought to know more about emotional trauma and manipulation. After 20 years in this field, I've helped numerous people escape the shackles of gaslighting. I have also been able to maintain my relationships with my husband, three lovely grown-up children, and two dogs. It has not always been easy, but there is nothing better than a healthy relationship—it helps your life blossom and makes everything less challenging.

In this book, we will review the signs of emotional abuse and manipulation, how you can easily detect the signs, how to fight back and break free when you are a victim of gaslighting, and how to deal with the aftermath of abuse so that you can live a healthier and happier life.

I want you to know that gaslighting doesn't need to be your way of life. You can break free from it. When you decide to gather the strength to break away, your torment can end! There is hope for you to heal and take back the life you've always known to be true. You are worthy of being loved. Your feelings and perceptions are not crazy; they are valid and need to be treated as such. You come first and shouldn't live by someone else's view of what is real.

So, are you ready to break free? Come with me as I take you through all you need to know about gaslighting and how to break free!

ONE

What is Gaslighting?

Being gaslighted isn't normal, and you should not settle for it if you find yourself in that situation. Many lives have been ruined or damaged due to the effects of gaslighting, but your life doesn't have to be one of them.

The phenomenon of gaslighting is the same all over the world. Gaslighters (the aggressors in these situations) are on a mission to manipulate and carry on emotional abuse toward others. Normally, an abuser would manipulate your beliefs and certain situations over and over again with the aim to trick you. This results in thoughts of mistrust and agony. Sadly, you will start to distrust your perceptions and memory as a result of this manipulation.

What is Gaslighting?

According to psychologists, "gaslighting" refers to a specific type of manipulation wherein the aggressor causes someone else and/or the people around them to question their own memory, reality, or perceptions. Gaslighters will make you believe that you are crazy and that you can't do anything on your own, making you feel dependent on them as a result. They will make you feel like you aren't intelligent enough to pass an exam, like you are the cause of everyone's problems, or like you're the worst person to be with.

When you are being gaslighted, you start losing the willingness and enthusiasm to be with people, and you begin to question your loyalty to family and friends. Through this constant manipulation, your self-confidence and self-esteem deteriorate over time.

Gaslighting is usually carried out by the people who know you very well, and it mostly occurs in personal relationships. It can range from an abusive spouse, or parents who want to keep you dependent on them, or even your boss constantly who constantly berates you and makes you feel incapable. The gaslighter may be your colleague at work who is jealous of your potential and begins taking advantage of you, or anybody close to you.

Gaslighting is a common tactic used by public figures as well. They have a collection of buzzwords and phrases like, "Stop being overdramatic, it's not a big deal," or, "Come on, I didn't mean it, you are just oversensitive," that is meant to shift the blame to you for accusing them. Even when the situation is highly sensitive, they will challenge your emotional strength. They can also deny ever having said or done something, despite any evidence to the contrary. Hearing such a phrase can take you down a rabbit hole where you think about when they said what they now deny. This feeling takes you to an unwanted solitude where you spiral alone with harmful thoughts. In reality, you are right and just getting mentally manipulated.

Almost all of us have been on the receiving end of some form of gaslighting at some point in our lives— not necessarily in a severe way, but it does happen more often than you might imagine. It is important to identify ways to shut gaslighting down and minimize the emotional and psychological impact it has on our lives. If gaslighting is left unattended to and unexamined, it can cause long-term damage to your mental health. In the next section, we will be looking at the origin of gaslighting to give us a better understanding of how it came to be.

The Origin of Gaslighting

As we discussed in the introduction, the term "gaslighting" originated from the play *Gas Light* in 1938 but wasn't popularized until the American film adaptation in 1944. The plot revolves around Jack

Manningham and his wife, Bella—the names were changed to Gregory and Paula in the American film adaptation.

In the film, Georgy began to drive Paula crazy by using various tricks and tactics, which resulted in her questioning her own perceptions and sanity. He started to adjust and control Paula's life. When she remarks about the changes happening in her life, he denies it. Slowly, Gregory makes her believe that she is going crazy. He carries out this scheme in order to claim his wife's inheritance. Later on, Paula realizes that she has been manipulated by her husband and has him arrested. She does this by letting Gregory believe that she's helping him escape, leading him into a trap set by the police.

This story is a prime example of both the effects of gaslighting on a victim as well as the tactics a gaslighter uses to manipulate the people around them.

Signs That You're Being Gaslighted

As a victim of gaslighting, you have been through a lot of emotional torment. A gaslighter does everything possible to make you feel like a loser who is too unstable to handle your emotions or your life. They get control over you and make you feel the way they want you to feel. But fear not; there are some notable signs that will help you to realize that you are being gaslighted. I will run through them so you can pick up on them and avoid being controlled by a gaslighter.

The common sights that you are being gaslighted are:

- You start second-guessing yourself. You will constantly criticize your thoughts, thinking you can never make important decisions on your own.
- You question your relationship(s). When you come to realize that your partner was not the person you thought they were, it can make you question your reality.
- You question your level of sensitivity. You will constantly ask yourself, "Am I too sensitive?" and will question your reactions to any given situation.
- You are filled with self-doubt. You start doubting your emotional health, memory, sanity, and your ability to function in society.
- You make excuses for someone's behavior. You always try to explain the behavior of another person by justifying and making excuses for their actions, even when they don't deserve it.
- You are quick to apologize for no reason. Even when you are sure about your innocence, you still feel sorry and

apologize. Your fear of making the situation worse and losing relationships causes you to take the blame for everything.

- You question your morality. You constantly think that you are not good enough and that no one loves you because you do not deserve love.

- You think that you can't do anything right. You blame yourself for every little mistake you make. You start believing that nothing can go right if you are involved.

- You start to lie to avoid put-downs and reality twists. When you don't want to discuss and admit the realities of your life, you start lying and making excuses to keep up the lie.

- You don't know how to express sadness. You know something is wrong and is making you terribly sad, but you cannot figure out what it is. You cannot even express your sadness to yourself.

- You blame yourself for not having a good relationship with others. Even when the other person is at fault and made a mistake, you blame yourself by saying things like, "Maybe I was wrong; that's why he did this to me."

- You start to make decisions with the

gaslighter in mind. Your thought process begins with whether they would accept your choice or not. You make decisions that can make them happy, not considering your happiness.

- You often feel hopeless and sad. The hopelessness makes you feel as if there is no light in your life, and that you will remain in the dark without someone to force you out.

- You feel unclear and vague about your thoughts, feelings, and emotions. You don't understand what is going on in your mind, and you cannot explain your thoughts in detail.

Signs/Characteristics of a Gaslighter

Now that you know the common signs of being gaslighted, it's important to know who the aggressor is. These parameters can help us to clearly know who the gaslighters are and what they do. The characteristics of gaslighters will let you know their tactics, the ways they manipulate you, control your emotions, and your ability to think on your own.

- **They use your fears against you.** Gaslighters often know how to control your fears and use them for their benefit.

They act charming in order to extract information from you but only intend to use your weaknesses to control you.

- **They tend to know everything about you.** Many gaslighters are those who claim to know everything about you and repeatedly tell you things like "I know you better than you know yourself," or "I know everything about you." If you deny them, they deny you in return by saying, "You are lying to yourself." This leads to you losing your confidence and self-esteem.

- **They make you question your sanity.** A person who is constantly abusing you wouldn't want you to be self-aware, so they challenge your perception whenever they can. Continuous manipulation tactics from a gaslighter can change the way you think. If you find yourself in an abusive relationship, it is easy for you to go along with the view of the abuser, which slowly changes the way you think and perceive things on your own.

- **They make you doubt yourself.** A gaslighter will take actions that lead you to doubt yourself and your abilities. They repeatedly deny your experiences and question your memories, and you start to doubt yourself eventually.

- **They drain your positive energy.** Gaslighters are fond of extracting positivity from you and try to fill you up with negative energy.

- **They make you start forgetting things.** Gaslighters can make you forget something they've said or done before. They make a commitment or a promise and then will deny it later when you try to bring it up again.

- **They make you lie.** Maybe you are not a person who lies, but a gaslighter is someone who makes you lie to avoid any verbal or physical abuse from them.

- **They make you question your decisions.** It is a trait of a gaslighter to challenge any and all decisions made by you. With them involved, you can never be confident in your decisions, and you will be weak in decision making over time.

- **They make excuses for what they don't want to accept.** For things that gaslighters don't want to accept, they will always make excuses and tend to redirect each suspicion. They do not want to face any inquiry and don't want to be accountable for anything.

- **They make you stay quiet and avoid people.** After being abused emotionally, the victim usually stops communicating with other people. They prefer to remain quiet and even stop sharing their experiences with others because of the traumatic experience or fear of retaliation.

- **They make you feel depressed.** A gaslighter can make anyone around them depressed. Questioning your sanity will make your mind tired, and your positive energy will get drained, leading to an onset of stress and depression. You may find yourself in a condition of hopelessness and unsolved chaos.

- **They constantly make demotivating comments.** Gaslighters often make demotivating comments to belittle and make you feel lesser than them. They will make comments like, "You are crazy" , "You can't do it right", "You are not made to do this work", "You are overreacting and being dramatic", or "You don't remember things right." All these statements are used by gaslighters to make their victims feel demotivated.

- **They want to be dominant over you.** Gaslighters don't let anybody else be in control. In fact, they always want to be dominant over you so that they can control you more easily.

All the above are characteristics of gaslighters. I have explained them so that you can easily identify a gaslighter when you come in contact with one. Gaslighting is done when a person has power over the other, and this is done all around us. It may not be easy given that gaslighters will do anything in their power to make you question your beliefs, but this knowledge will help you become more aware and less susceptible to their tricks.

TWO

Who is a Suspect?

G aslighting is a psychological term that refers to the particular behavior of a person—behavior by which one person manipulates the perception of reality for another person. That person is a victim of gaslighting. The victim suffers because of the gaslighter. So, who is a suspect? Whom should we say is manipulating the emotional rights of others? There are many examples of gaslighting. Let's explore some of these examples to better understand what we are dealing with.

It is commonly believed that gaslighting can't be suspected and identified. Only a person who suffers from it knows what they are going through. But the aim of this section of the book is to let you know what type of person may be manipulating you. Knowing common examples of who the typical aggressors are will make it easy for you to widen your understanding of gaslighting, and who to avoid if they begin to show signs of manipulation.

At Work: Boss, Colleagues, & Business Partners

Workplaces and gaslighting have a deep connection with each other. Gaslighting in the workplace can happen in many ways. Most gaslighting in this setting is done by an aggressor who is in a higher position of power than their victim. This can range from a boss, or an employer, or even the head of a particular department. But this doesn't stop with people in power. Gaslighting can easily occur to anyone at work —even between two coworkers who work at the same level under the same supervisor.

If gaslighting occurs where there is a hierarchy between employees, it is clearly an act of abuse happening through the use of power, and this should be reported by the victim. Employees, bosses, or any other person can easily manipulate others and make them question the realities. If you experience this sort of behavior at work, the HR department is the best place to turn to for help in the first instance.

Gaslighting at work commonly has a motivation behind it. It could be that the aggressor feels that someone is easy to victimize, or that the victim already devalues and does not like themselves. For example, a typical target for workplace gaslighting will say things like, "I am not good at this job", or "I'll be stuck at this job forever, there's no hope for me." These statements invite a gaslighter to come and tell you the same things to reaffirm what the victim already believes.

According to Australian psychologist Amberley Meredith, "Gaslighters have a very domineering personality." Moreover, she says that gaslighting happens both horizontally (between coworkers) and vertically (between boss and workers) (Neilson, 2019).

Gaslighting in the workplace often takes place when one person knows the weak spots of another. They are not just narcissists who want to be praised and want everyone to think that they are the best at their job. They are the ones who are cruel in their intentions and aim to use weak spots of others against them.

Listed below are various examples of gaslighting in the workplace. My aim is to clarify the situations you could face at work. This will give you a heads-up and let you know when a suspect is trying to gaslight you. Please note that in the examples below, and other places in this book, I may refer to a fictional person as a he, she, they, or them. This is purely arbitrary and does not imply that a man or woman is more or less likely to be on the giving or receiving end of gaslighting.

- **Example 1:** At the workplace, an employee is asked to perform an urgent task. She pauses her current task (we'll call this Task X) and starts working on the new one (which we'll call Task Y). After completing the task, she reports back to the Boss with the results. The Boss then responds, "I asked you to complete Task X, why are you wasting your time on Task Y?". She listens to this remark and gets flustered and tries to defend herself. What is the consequence then? The Boss then retorts with, "Don't you think that you are being over-dramatic? You need to calm down." She, in return, might become confused about her position, questioning whether or not she was in the wrong or if the Boss was. If the Boss is successful in these tactics, she might blame herself.

- **Example 2:** An employee is told that he will be given a bonus, promotion, or get a raise after a certain amount of time when he makes certain deadlines and performs well. The employee works hard to meet the Boss' requirements to get the raise. When he goes to the Boss with an achievement, the Boss says something like, "When did I say that I will promote you? I only said that I will think about it based on your performance, which is lacking right now."

Some employees may feel depressed after hearing things like this.

- **Example 3:** Sometimes, when some employee wants you to help them with a task that they are doing, they will butter you up by giving you compliments, praising your abilities, and bragging about your talent in front of you and other employees. You get confused because they have never complimented you in the past. In fact, they've frequently said that you were unqualified and terrible at your job. This is how they manipulate, both into doing what they want and challenging your perception of past events. This causes you to start doubting yourself and distrusting compliments from others.

- **Example 4:** Let's say that you have two workers who start at the same level—then, one of them gets promoted. The one with the promotion will begin saying things that will lower the confidence of the other. They will say things like, "I think the boss is not satisfied with your performance," or "I heard that you were not in that email; I think the Boss doesn't trust you with information yet," or "I don't think you will be getting promoted until the end of this year, if ever." All these lines are tactics used to kill the morale of the victim employee.

- **Example 5:** Sometimes, an employee will discriminate on the basis of race or sex. The aggressor will make inappropriate comments, and then deny the victim's allegations when the victim reports them to HR or to their employer. Depending on the work environment, the claims will end up brushed under the rug, leaving the victim disillusioned and right back at square one.

All of the above examples depict how individuals in the workplace get manipulated and mentally tortured by bosses or coworkers. This type of environment isn't healthy and can result in mental fatigue. The victim loses interest in their job and cannot become satisfied because they are in a situation where they question their abilities and sanity. If you find yourself in this situation and have the ability to get out of it, you should do so. You don't have to put up with this treatment in the workplace.

Family: Parents, Grandparents, & Siblings

Living in a family composed of people who claim to love you and care for you is beautiful and should not be taken for granted. But not all families are meant to be perfect. There are victims of gaslighting who are being manipulated by their very own family members.

Unfortunately, it is not always the case that only one member of the family is a gaslighter. There can be multiple people within one family tormenting one victim. In a family dynamic, the most aggressor is the parents/guardians gaslighting their child. This is because half of the world view and life experience of children comes from their parents. Also, parents think that they have every right to treat their child however they want. They forget to build the emotional health and self-esteem of their children and end up ruining their confidence and life through their actions, which can end up being emotional abuse. Whether this behavior is conscious or not depends on the situation.

Children are affected by manipulation from their parents because their worldview gets influenced by what their parents say and do. Children will often face a situation where they are blamed and even punished for their mistakes. Sometimes parents blame their children for their own mistakes, which they refuse to accept.

There are also times where grandparents become aggressors in emotional abuse. They often make their grandchildren feel like they are nothing, and they begin to question their existence. Gaslighting can also take place between siblings, where one sibling tries to manipulate the other one and bring their confidence down. Gaslighting among siblings is easier to control, but it becomes difficult to control this dynamic within parent/child relationships.

Gaslighting in the family is more difficult to recognize than other instances of gaslighting. The age factor makes the older aggressor more dominant over others, and this allows them to more easily gaslight their younger victims. A gaslighter is always superior to the one who is being gaslighted. For instance, if parents or grandparents interfere in the lives of their children and challenge their reality, the children will suffer and lose their interest in life.

Family gaslighters have an easier time gaslighting their victims than a boss gaslighting their workers. A gaslighter in the family has the ability to attack the family member on any front. To get a better understanding of this, we will discuss examples of family gaslighting below. In these examples, we will show how a child can be manipulated and challenged by their parents and grandparents.

- **Example 1:** There is a child who needs to get to school on time, and the parent delays the child, so they get to school late. The parent will blame their child for being late to school and refuse to accept that they caused the delay themselves. They say, "You will be late for school because you stayed up late playing on your computer! Why don't you just behave yourself and do what you're told?" This type of statement will cause a child to doubt their punctuality and reliability. They will believe that it's they're fault, even when they aren't at fault.

- **Example 2:** Parents are known to let children know their limits, and that crossing them can result in the child being punished. But sometimes, parents can become violent in the process of reinforcing the boundaries of their children. They do not want their rules to be broken, and this makes them gradually turn into gaslighters without knowing.

- **Example 3:** In this scenario, a parent promises to reward something to their child if they do something they are told to do. When the child eventually does it and asks their parents to fulfill their promise, the parent will deny what they said by claiming that they never made any promises. This causes a child to mistrust their family, whom they had no reason to distrust in the past. Also, their confidence wanes, and they start to question their memory after denial from their parents.

- **Example 4:** Some parents will call their child by harsh nicknames, which devalue or demotivate them. They do not realize what damage those words can cause to the child. They keep on with the name-calling, and later, they claim that it was a joke and that nothing was serious about it. They might say, "I didn't mean to make my child feel down; it was just a joke." "Oh my! My child is oversensitive". This kills a child inwardly, especially when it comes from their parents.

At first, it seems very unlikely for parents to understand their children's emotions. They devalue their children's emotions by claiming that they are pretending or over-dramatizing their acts. In their opinion, their child only wants to seek attention. But this is not true; children show real emotions and tend to be more honest with how they feel than adults. It is the parents who don't understand how their children feel.

Similarly, gaslighting among siblings is very common. In this case, one sibling tries to manipulate the other. Sometimes they turn into a narcissist and keep on demoralizing their sibling, which creates a feeling of being a loser in the victim. The victim loses interest in their personality and questions their abilities and sanity.

Relationship: Between Partners

Gaslighting is a form of psychological manipulation that has made its place in relationships between romantic partners. Emotional abuse is reported to be in the highest ratio among life partners these days. This refers to the tactics used by one partner to show power, to gain control, and to cause emotional damage to another. In this relationship dynamic, if one person wants to get control over another, they use techniques that make the whole relationship toxic by acting abusively to the other.

The situation in which two parties share their lives and know everything about each other is more open to attacks from one of the partners. It is easy for one of them to manipulate others by making them question their perception of reality. Gaslighting among partners often takes place when one partner loses interest in the other partner, when their chemistry doesn't match anymore, and/or when they discover issues and faults in the other.

To the outside world, two people in a relationship might seem loving and intimate, but this is not always true. A type of manipulation rules out true love and affection. There are many consequences associated with gaslighting within a relationship. Some partners choose to leave the toxic relationship as they value their mental health more, while others choose to stay in a toxic relationship (due to a lack of self-esteem, fear for their physical well-being, etc.), allowing their partner to manipulate them.

Some examples of gaslighting taking place within a relationship are as follows:

- **Example 1:** When the controlling partner makes a commitment with the other partner. Let's say that they were supposed to do something together on Saturday. When Saturday comes around, and the victim tries reminding their partner (the gaslighter) about what they were supposed to do together, the gaslighter might say, "No, silly. I said Sunday and not Saturday." The victim then becomes confused, thinking about their memory and feeling that they remembered wrong or misheard. The effects make them start questioning their own memory.
- **Example 2:** Sometimes, one partner will make the other feel embarrassed for no reason. They deny their own words or claim that they did not mean what the other partner perceived. Let's take the conversation below as an example:
- *Partner 1:* "I just spoke to my mum, and she and my dad have agreed to see you this

weekend. They are so excited to finally meet you."

- ***Partner 2:*** "I told you that we needed to wait a little more before involving your family.

- ***Partner 1:*** "We actually talked about it, and you seemed excited to meet them."

- ***Partner 2:*** "Yes, I do, but isn't it too early? I am happy to meet them, but I also said to give this a little more time. You are always forcing things, and if things go wrong, you are the cause of it."

Where does this type of conversation lead to? It makes Partner 1 feel stupid and question their decision to set up a meeting with the parents. This makes Partner 1 question their memory and sanity.

- **Example 3:** Another example of gaslighting among couples can be when one partner wants to take complete control over the other. They want to control their thoughts and don't want others to tell them about their actions, whether they're right or wrong. In this type of gaslighting, controlling partners do not let the other see their friends and family. They think that these people will change their minds about them and open their eyes to see what the victim isn't initially seeing. They fear that the victim will end up leaving them if they get to recover from the abuse. They might love their partner, but their possessiveness makes them turn to emotional abuse. If care is not taken, this type of gaslighting can often lead to physical abuse.

- **Example 4:** Our final case is when one partner reacts to statements or questions from the other partner with lies. This happens when a partner claims the other partner said something when, in reality, it is all a lie. Let's take a look at the conversation below to see how it work:

- *Partner 1:* "Do you remember that you asked me to use your credit card whenever I want to? I just saw a leather bag that I wanted to buy for so long."

- *Partner 2:* "I doubt if I actually said that. I just can't remember when I did."

The lying partner will go on and on to spin lies about how they asked, and when they asked, creating fictitious scenes just to justify the lies. This type of gaslighting will lead the victim partner to doubt themselves and allow the gaslighter to have control over them, their life, feelings, and possessions.

THREE

What Makes Them Do It?

By now, you should know what gaslighting is and how it is used by manipulators. Gaslighting is one person's attempt to control the reality of another. It is a type of emotional abuse that is done to make a targeted individual question their reality.

In this chapter, we will be looking at what makes a gaslighter do the things they do. What are the reasons that make them want to have control over others, and why do they make it a goal to make the victim question their reality, memory, and sanity?

Obviously, a gaslighter wasn't born that way. There are some factors that have taken place that make them want to manipulate and control others. The personality of the gaslighter and the way they were brought up by their family can factor into this.

The reasons which make individual gaslight others will be discussed as we proceed.

Why Do People Gaslight?

There are a lot of reasons and factors that make a gaslighter want to manipulate others. Many people—not just gaslighters—have insecurities about their identity, as they don't want to show their real selves to the world or have not explored their identity. This results in them knowing little or nothing about who they are and who they wish to be. This is why they tend to present their false self in front of the world. They keep a mask on their face to show society and are more likely to challenge the reality of other people rather than doing any kind of self-reflection.

Gaslighters don't know or understand their reality, so they find it difficult to be honest. They want other people to carry their insecurities with them. But the reason they do this is that they do not want to face themselves. This can often stem from a personality disorder that they suffer from. They just offload their emotional stress over for other people to deal with. They want to spend their life with lies all around them. This state is known as psychopathy. Psychopathy is a pattern of unprompted lies—also known as pathological lying—and a condition that makes people manipulate others.

Another reason people gaslight is to gain power

over others. The thought of controlling other people will come to their mind because of their antisocial personality or because of them being a narcissist. They want to feel special and want others to praise them for their uniqueness. Being a sadist can also make people gaslight. Sadism is an emotional feeling in which individuals want to cause harm and pain to other people around them.

Sometimes when someone wants to get something badly enough, they manipulate others to get what they want. This condition is known as Machiavellianism, which refers to cold and dry acts from an individual in which they manipulate other people to achieve their goals. This condition arises when they are unable to achieve something in their life. This one is also the main reason behind gaslighting.

People who grow up facing family problems are more likely to gaslight others. They didn't receive much love and praise while growing up and, in the process, lost their identity. Rather than finding themselves, they choose to violate the feelings and realities of others. From this, we can see that people who have a disturbing childhood are more likely to gaslight others. They try to have control over others and want to get praise from them because they didn't get it while growing up.

In summary, the reasons why most people gaslight are as follows:

- They want to be in control of others and exert their power on them.
- They were probably raised by parents who were gaslighters. Many children suffer from being gaslighted and end up turning into a gaslighter who, in turn, ruins the lives of other people around them. Such children learn this from their parents and don't see the act as wrong.
- They feel they have a right to impose their thoughts and beliefs on other people and can show their power upon them.

These examples are not a formulaic checklist and do not reflect on all people who have had rough childhoods or haven't been able to get what they want. But they do tend to pop up frequently in gaslighters, so it doesn't hurt to be aware of these trends.

Types of Gaslighting

The aim of gaslighters is to make their victims have self-doubt, and eventually make victims believe that what the abuser says is always true no matter how ridiculous it sounds or appears. Whether a gaslighter callously attacks the victim's mental health or character, or rains insults on his victim, it is still gaslighting done in different ways. It all depends on the abuser's style of gaslighting and how effective the type of gaslighting he uses.

This brings us to the types of gaslighting. There are different ways in which gaslighters abuse their victims. Some gaslighters may intentionally abuse their victims, while others don't intentionally do it. We will be exploring the different types of gaslighting below.

Conscious Gaslighting

Conscious gaslighting is usually intentional. A gaslighter intentionally makes other people victims of their manipulation. They knowingly make people question their reality and memory. This type of gaslighting is dangerous and can be damaging to the victim. Among the types of gaslighting, conscious gaslighting is the most abusive and inimical one.

This type of gaslighter knows what they are doing to victims, yet they still go ahead to control their thoughts, damage their personality, and achieve their goals. These types of gaslighters don't feel sorry for manipulating the people close to them and will still find excuses to shift the blame to their victims. This is usually why some survivors of emotional abuse have damaging and long-lasting symptoms.

Individuals who suffer from antisocial personality disorder are among the common cases of people who strive to keep control over someone in their life.

This need to have control over other's lives causes them to gaslight others. The disorder lets people manipulate others by imposing their power on them, and they tend to manipulate people with their actions and words. Wanting everyone under their control is their main aim. All that they want and do is intentional. They know what they feel, what they are about to do, and what the results will be. Still, they choose to gaslight others and ruin someone else's perspective.

Another type of personality disorder that often appears in gaslighters is Authoritarian personality, which makes the individual believe that their own perceptions are the only ones that matter. They don't value other people's beliefs and perspectives. This type of person always wants the people around them to believe that they are right and that everyone around them is wrong. They try to convince others of their reality, which might not be true to other people. They don't even have an idea of their own reality and identity, yet they disregard other people's perceptions and values. To them, "If it seems true and right to me, then it should be true and right to others." They do not feel the need to respect other people's perspectives and refuse to analyze whether or not their line of thinking is right or wrong.

People with the Authoritarian personality are fond of manipulating others with their beliefs when they don't value theirs and end up making them silent.

Victims will feel tortured and question their abilities to understand and comprehend things.

For a better understanding of people with this type of personality that uses the conscious gaslighting, let's take a look at some example scenarios:

A husband is on a business trip far away from his home. He and his wife have a joint bank account. He withdraws cash from an ATM and turns his phone off. The wife immediately starts calling him, demanding to know what the withdrawal was for since they didn't agree to do such a thing, but she didn't receive a response. After many hours, the wife gets hold of him and asks, "What were you doing while you were out of reach, and why did you withdraw cash from the ATM?"

The husband then replies, "I needed to pay the taxi bill, and my phone was unreachable because I was at a place where the phone signal is bad. Wow, I am so amazed that you called me just to fight! Is this how you treat people you love? I think you are going through some kind of depression. I am so far from home, and you just wanted to pick a fight with me because of a withdrawal I made?"

The wife will feel bad for going all out on him and might end up saying, "Oh! I am sorry. I didn't mean to fight with you, honey." Even though she hasn't done anything wrong, she becomes apologetic.

This is a case of intentional gaslighting on the part of the husband. He lied to his wife about why he needed to withdraw money and covered his flaws blaming his wife. This can cause a feeling of depression and doubtfulness in the wife, and she will feel sorry for no reason. Moreover, he diverted his wife's attention from his behavior and made her feel guilty instead.

Another example of intentional gaslighting is when a boss denies what he promised to his employee, and makes the employee feel guilty about asking for the promised thing. For instance, a boss asks his employee to take charge of a contract he had wanted to get for so long. He then promised the employee a salary raise and promotion if the contract goes well. The employee works hard to make the contract successful.

After the business deal is closed, he reports to the boss and reminds him of the salary raise, and promotion promised to him. The boss denies by saying, "Oh! I don't remember saying anything like that. I think you must be mistaken. You have earned this project, but your performance does not deserve promotion right now, work harder, and you will get it."

This can make the employee feel so disheartened. Because of this, they will get confused and start doubting themselves. Moreover, this intentional gaslighting done by the boss makes the employee question their abilities and start feeling unmotivated to work harder.

Semi-Intentional Gaslighting

This is a type of gaslighting which is done intentionally, but without the knowledge of the impact, it has on another person. Semi-intentional gaslighting is done to keep people away so as not to hurt them or to manipulate them. But it is still a form of gaslighting, so it has a negative impact on other people. A person who performs acts of semi-intentional gaslighting might know that the other person will understand and will act accordingly after listening to their response. This is a sort of tactic used by people to push others away from them.

Semi-intentional gaslighting makes people confused about their emotions. Let's say, for example, that there is a man who is sad and wants to be alone with his sadness. He does not want anybody to share in his grief and sorrow. So, when his wife comes and sees him alone and wallowing in his emotions, she asks for the reason. The husband answers, "Nothing is wrong. I'm totally fine." This is obviously a lie, and this leaves the wife feeling confused as to why he's lying; so, she leaves him alone.

If the husband told her what he is feeling or going through, the problem could be solved easily. But since the husband did not want to show his pain to another person, he preferred to lie, which left his wife in confusion and left him further in his depression. This is an example of someone gaslighting to create distance between themselves and the people around them. Semi-intentional gaslighting does not create long-lasting effects for the victim, but it still has an effect on others in the moment.

Another scenario could be when someone gaslights without realizing that what they're doing is wrong. Maybe some people have gone through gaslighting by their parents, and they end up doing the same thing with their children. These people justify their actions saying things like, "This is how I was raised, and it is totally fine. My kid needs to toughen up just like I had to." They don't know the impact the act has on others by doing this. They keep on manipulating others without realizing that what they are doing is wrong and damaging to the person simply because they didn't understand that it was wrong when they received the same treatment.

Unintentional Gaslighting

This type of gaslighting is not a regular or conscious pattern of behavior. It often happens by accident, like someone not knowing that they are manipulating others. This type of gaslighting does not cause lasting harm or become a problem for others. Some people use intentional gaslighting and are aware of their wrong behavior, while some use semi-intentional gaslighting and are only partially aware of their actions. But a large number of people in the world use unintentional gaslighting tactics accidentally in their everyday life. These people don't intentionally gaslight others, so this form of gaslighting is less harmful than the other two forms.

Let's take a look at a few different scenarios to help us better understand this type of gaslighting.

A mother is in the kitchen preparing a mushroom salad for the whole family. Her son enters and says, "Mum, I don't like salad." His mother answers him with, "Don't say that. Salad is so yummy, and you love it, remember?" Her son nods and agrees reluctantly. Later, the mother realizes that she has imposed something on her child that conflicts with his reality. He doesn't like salad at all, but in order to convince him to eat salad, she contradicted his reality. The mother didn't intentionally confuse her child, but some confusion has already taken place by gaslighting him to believe he likes salad.

A child sitting in a living room says to his parents that he does not want to go to grandma's place because he does not like being there. In order for the father to ease the situation and to change the mind of a child, he might say, "You like being there honey, don't say that!" This is how parents tend to manipulate the reality of their kids. In this example, the intention of parents was not spiteful, but gaslighting still occurred. The parent has devalued and disturbed the opinion of their child, which caused confusion in their child about reality.

Another example is a girl who has a disorder that makes her seem abnormal to people. She doesn't care about her appearance and goes shopping with her mother. People keep on staring at her and passing comments about her appearance. There was one person in particular who kept staring at her. She asked them, "Why are you staring at me like this, stop doing this!" The person replied, "No! You took it wrong. I was staring at you because you look so pretty, don't be oversensitive". Here, unintentional gaslighting took place. The person made a comment on her beauty when he knew that wasn't why he was staring at her. In addition, the person also made mention of the girl being overly sensitive. This can make the girl start doubting herself.

No matter the form, unintentional gaslighting is still not acceptable as it still causes confusion and doubt for victims.

FOUR

When Do the Lights Flicker?

B y now, you should know that gaslighting is a form of mental and emotional abuse in which other people and their feelings are manipulated by an aggressor, which we refer to as a gaslighter. It leads to abusive relationships, no matter who the people are and what type of relationship they have. Gaslighting is a type of emotional abuse in which the abuser targets a person and makes them question their reality and challenge their memory. Gaslighting leads to feelings of stress and depression in the victim.

In this chapter, we will be looking at the symptoms and signs related to gaslighting. There must be some set standard in which we can agree that gaslighting is taking place, so we need to cover these areas to be sure of what you are experiencing or have experienced. The techniques and tactics used by gaslighters to manipulate people will also be discussed in this chapter.

Principal Techniques of a Gaslighter

After analyzing the types of gaslighting, it is essential for you to know about the ways a person manipulates others through specific techniques. These techniques are used by a gaslighter to hide the realities of their victims. They don't want the victim to realize the truth they have been hiding from them and will use some techniques to cover it up. The common techniques for gaslighting are:

Withholding: This is a technique in which the abuser refuses to listen and share their emotions with others. There is no understanding of the truth with people who use this technique. To hide their own truths, they tend to lie. They refuse to listen to what they are being told and don't want to understand others. For instance, "Come on, I am not ready to listen again to the crap you said last night." Or "I am not listening to you, stop messing with my head." These statements can make the people listening fall prey to manipulation because victims will feel that the gaslighter is not interested in them, and they will do anything to get them interested.

Countering: This is another technique of gaslighting in which the abuser creates a situation where the victim questions their memory. Gaslighters who use this technique will tell their victims that they don't remember saying or doing certain things, even when the victim has a very good memory and/or proof. For example, "Remember when you forgot what we were talking about that last time, you are getting old even at 22". Or "You do not think things through correctly, and you always remember things wrong."

Blocking and Diverting: Gaslighters use this technique when they want to divert the attention of the victim from any matter or thought. They change the situation or can claim that what the victim is saying is not right at all. They tend to change the subject to question the thoughts of the victim and take control of the conversation, and oftentimes, they succeed in doing this. For example, "Wait, who gave you this stupid idea?" Or, "Do you remember, you did the same thing!" Or "You are hurting me now. How do you think I feel?"

Trivializing: This technique is used to discourage the thoughts and emotions of a particular victim. They will convince the victim that what they are thinking is wrong or that they're being too sensitive. They don't see any reason for the victim to feel what they are feeling. Through this technique, a gaslighter makes the victim believe that their thoughts, emotions, and needs are not important. This leads the victim to feel guilty about their own emotions and to doubt whether or not they are being too sensitive. For example, "It was not like that, you are just overly sensitive." Or, "Are you going to let something this small come between us like this?" Or, "We need to move on, stop overthinking about it. It's not an issue."

Forgetting and Denial: Through this technique, the gaslighter claims that they forgot about a past event, or about something either you or they said. They may even deny the occurrence of any past event even if they remember it, and instead tell the victim that they forgot. It might be a promise they made to the victim or harsh words that they "didn't mean". For example, "I don't remember something like that happened." Or, "Was I there when all this was happening?" Or, "I don't have to take this; I am sure I didn't say that."

Also, some gaslighters enjoy mocking and discouraging the feelings and emotions of their victims. They gaslight others based on their wrongdoings and misperceptions. A gaslighter may decide to use one or more of the above techniques to make victims doubt their feelings, emotions, and memories. This art in psychology makes the victim believe that they must keep quiet, lest they be proven wrong again. The victim will become too timid to speak up because there is this fear of making another mistake. With this, they might go into continuous confusion and remember events incorrectly. In some cases, the abuser accuses the victim of being a gaslighter. They say that other people are gaslighting them when, in reality, they are the true gaslighters.

What Does an Abuser Do to Gaslight Others?

Gaslighting is an act that can be done by anyone without the victim realizing what they are doing. Gaslighting is known to be a common tactic used by narcissists, abusers, dictators, and cult leaders. This means everyone who sees themselves as dominant and better than others can gaslight them for no reason. Gaslighting is done slowly and over time. In fact, it is so gradual that victims often don't realize how much they have been ruined mentally and emotionally by these tactics. The fact is that a gaslighter can have a very charming and confident personality. They gaslight the victim so silently that the victim believes that the gaslighter could never do something so terrible. They start second-guessing the actions of the gaslighter. Abusers then use some techniques to prove what the victim feels about them is right.

As a result, a victim starts to ignore their own feelings and gut instincts. They begin to believe what the abuser wants them to believe.

Later in this chapter, we will highlight some tactics used by gaslighters. You will see what the symptoms are and signs a gaslighter shows. This will help you to recognize the gaslighters around you and will help to remain safe from such abusive people.

They keep lying. Firstly, people who gaslight others lie a lot. They always know when and why they are lying. It is not a problem for them because they tell lies with such ease and without any form of guilt. They lie to the victim with such flippancy that it becomes second nature. They lie with such an experience that even if a victim provides proof of their dishonesty, the abuser will still claim that their lie is the truth and will make the victim question their accusations. Victims will start to doubt their own reality, and this is a first step an abuser may take to make them question their perceptions. This starts an abusive pattern in which the victim starts doubting their own thoughts and memory. After constant lies, victims will go deep into a spiral of self-doubt, and this is exactly what gaslighters want.

They attack what you love. Gaslighters have this attitude of discrediting things and people in the victim's life. They want to take cherished things and people away from the victims to make them feel unsure about everything. They use the things which are closest to the victim against them. For example, if someone loves their job and enjoys doing it, the abuser will start to find issues that will make them want to quit that job. Or if someone has a loving spouse, a gaslighter may plant the seed of mistrust in them and cause confusion in the marriage. All these tactics used by abusers make the victims fall into chaos about the things and people they love, and they start to question themselves about their perception and ability to keep people and something close to them. They will end up blaming themselves for not being worthy of the relationships and joys around them.

Deny, deny, deny. Even when victims know and remember what an abuser said in the past, the abuser will simply deny the things they say. First, they will deny it and then ask the victim to prove that incident and conversation if it really happened. They know that the victim only has a slight memory of the conversation and that they do not remember the whole event. By this point, the victim starts to doubt their memory by thinking that the abuser may be right. "Maybe they didn't say what I remembered, and I must be wrong at this place." Due to this, victims will question their memory and reality and believe themselves to be at fault.

Discrediting. Discrediting is what is done by gaslighters in two ways. In the first case, they will say they are worried about the victim in front of other people. They are worried because they think that the victim does not know how to handle a particular thing, as they are unstable and seem to be incapable of handling their own life. This way, they will discredit the victim. The victim will feel bad and confused because the abuser always mentions their insecurities and faults in public with sympathy and by showing care towards them. They will feel that they are not worthy of doing anything good and become dependent on the abuser as a result.

Another way abusers discredit victims is by making them believe some lie about people close to the victims in order to isolate them and keep them away from people that care about them. A gaslighter tries to discredit the friends of the victim by implying that the friends talked about them wrongly. Although this is a blatant lie, they still imply that everything others say is a lie and will make people around the victim believe them eventually. Also, the victim will feel that only the abuser is loyal to them and is the only person who really cares, believing every other person to be a liar and cheat on them.

Shifting blame. This tactic is used by gaslighters to shift their responsibilities to others so that they won't be blamed for anything. They will change the whole conversation in a way that the victim will end up apologizing for something they didn't do or say. They might also claim that the victim is responsible for their wrong behavior and that it is the victim who makes them lie in the first place. For example, when a person is too sensitive about any subject, the gaslighter will make it obvious that they are a hero, and the sensitive one is a victim. They end up shifting the blame on others, allowing them to have the upper hand.

They show love and flattery. This is another technique used by gaslighters, shower their victims with love and care when they are low or hurt because of something. They show constant love and flattery in the beginning, only to tear them down in the long run. It is a technique they use to gain the trust of their victims. Abusers may derive pleasure in doing this. The show of love and flattery usually brings uneasiness to the victim. They don't feel happy deep down by the attitude of the abuser. But the abuser is getting the victim used to getting torn down and then getting lifted up with flattery and love. This attitude of abusers makes the victim believe that the abusers are loyal to them. This is why victims cannot figure out what is really happening to them in the beginning.

Reframing. This is when the abuser turns around a past incident in their favor, leaving all the blame for everyone but themselves. They will try to find the fault of victims even when all the fault is theirs, and they often succeed in doing this. They may claim that they did not shove the victim and imply that the victim gets triggered easily. Now the victim will be confused, thinking it is their fault they got triggered and not the abuser's fault for shoving them in the first place.

Constantly calling you crazy. When a person who is in an abusive relationship and constantly gets attacked with emotional abuse focuses on building their sanity, the abuser will question their sanity. The gaslighter is aware that the victim is trying to find clarity for certain events and their perceptions, so, in order to disrupt what is going on, they call the victim crazy or try to change the new perception the victim is forming. Gaslighters may also convince other people about the victim's craziness. Because of this, if a victim would ever think to approach those people to seek help against the abuser, they would not be taken seriously.

Positive reinforcement. Another tactic used by gaslighters is to show a soothing attitude towards a person, and yet still manipulate them in the end. They use positive comments and compliments on the victim. Hearing the nice comments about themselves from an abuser will make them believe that everything is fine and that no one is doing them wrong. Gaslighters know that everyone has their limits, so they try to reel the person by showing kindness and love for them until they finally give in.

Their actions do not match their words. Gaslighters don't always do what they say they will do, and what they say often contradicts their actions. This is why their words shouldn't be given much importance. Still, by using some tricks, they let their victim believe all that they say to be fact.

How to Know if a Person is Being Gaslighted

People who are on the receiving end of mental and emotional abuse feel some symptoms or see signs that let them know that they are being gaslighted. It is important for everyone to check the signs that may arise and to know how to tell when you are being gaslighted.

As we discussed before, gaslighting is done so slowly and gradually that victims will not realize what is happening to them in the moments. To be safe, you can check to see if you notice any of the signs listed below. If yes, it is very likely that you are being gaslighted. If they are not, then it is a good sign; but you should be aware that gaslighters are everywhere, and you should be careful not to fall victim.

The common signs to note within yourself are:

- You continuously second-guess yourself. You find it hard to make decisions. Even if you make a decision, you do not believe it to be right and continue to doubt your own decision-making abilities.
- You filter your choices through the lens of the gaslighter and put the approval of the gaslighter before your choices and happiness. You become apologetic. You are ready to apologize for everything, even if you know that you didn't make a mistake.
- You start doubting your perception of reality and keep on questioning yourself about your personality and how valid your emotions are. Sometimes, when you think too much

about your reality, you become oversensitive and begin giving in to gaslighters.

- You feel you are not good enough and that people do not like you. All these thoughts will make you believe you are actually not good enough, even if they are implanted in your mind by the gaslighter.
- You become completely dependent on the gaslighter. You distance yourself from your loved ones and become overly attached and reliant on the gaslighter.
- If you were jolly, joyful, and full of life, you find that you've turned into a joyless, unhappy, and unsatisfied person without any reasonable explanation.
- You want to remain silent and fear to "speak up". Because of your past experience with a gaslighter, you believe that if you share your opinions and emotions, you will feel worse; so, you choose to remain silent.
- You usually sense that something is wrong but cannot identify what it is. This is because the gaslighter constantly confuses you and makes you doubt your emotions.
- You wonder why you don't feel happy most times, even when there are so many good things happening in your life.

- You tend to lie out of fear. You lie because you fear being called wrong, criticized, or getting attacked verbally. To avoid these situations, you form a pattern of pathological lying.
- You always think twice before bringing up any seemingly innocent topics or conversations.
- Before your partner comes back home, you make a checklist and analyze your actions from the whole day. You do this to put yourself in check and avoid doing anything wrong.
- You always talk to the people close to the abuser because you fear that talking to them directly will upset them. For example, a wife may call her husband's secretary to find out when he will be returning home because she is afraid it might make him upset if she calls him directly.
- You always think that you are not capable of doing anything productive and belong to the group of losers who won't make anything of themselves.

All of these signs show that you could be the victim of gaslighting. It is essential for everyone to try to recognize the signs in order to avoid being gaslighted by the people around you.

Gaslighting: The Narcissist's Favorite Tool

Gaslighting is a tool often used by narcissists to instill an extreme sense of confusion and anxiety in their victims. The way they use this technique is similar to the methods used in interrogation, brainwashing, and torture—tactics only used in psychological warfare by law enforcement, intelligence operative, and other special forces.

Narcissists usually suffer from a disorder called Narcissistic Personality Disorder (NPD). People suffering from this disorder often find themselves involved in activities based around manipulating people, abusing their partners, families, or friends. For certain types of abusers, it is difficult to point out the reason that makes them abuse others; they can't help but do it.

Translating A Narcissist's Language

Narcissistic abusers use certain tactics to devalue and manipulate their victims behind closed doors, refusing to let anyone on the outside know their true intentions. These people lack empathy, have an unearned sense of superiority, an uncontrollable love, and care for themselves, and they never think of others.

Narcissists use tactics like stonewalling (a refusal to communicate or cooperate), emotional abuse, projection, and manipulation of others just to be in control of their victim's life. If you have ever been in a relationship with a manipulative or toxic person, you know that they use language differently from others.

The common phrases we use every day in conversations have a different meaning in context when said by an abusive person, and vice versa. When dealing with someone that lacks empathy, has a high sense of entitlement, and a superior need to bring other people down, you will have conversations that are meant to divert and terrorize you psychologically. To decode the language of a narcissist, you need to listen closely to their actions and less to their words. When you can translate the narcissist's words into their actual meaning, you will see how disturbing the results are. Below are common phrases narcissists use for their victims, and their translations:

- **Phrase:** I am sorry you feel this way.
- **Translation:** I am sorry, but not sorry. We should just get this over with, so I can continue with my abusive behavior. I am sorry for getting caught and not for doing what I did. I am sorry for being held accountable and not for how you feel. How you feel is invalid to me because I

should be in control of how you feel, regardless of the effect on you.

- **Phrase:** You are overreacting/being oversensitive.
- **Translation:** What I am doing to you is the right thing and shouldn't be seen as a big deal. You are reacting normally to an immense amount of gaslighting, and you are catching on to my behavior. I will gaslight you more so that you can second-guess yourself. A key to keeping you compliant is by emotionally invalidating you. As long as you don't trust yourself, you will work very hard to minimize, rationalize, and deny my abuse. As you continue working hard to please me, I will continue to reap the benefits without facing any consequences.
- **Phrase:** You're crazy.
- **Translation:** I am good at creating confusion to trigger you, and I like it when you react. I will accuse you as the crazy one since no one will believe you or listen to what you have to say. They already see you as unstable and bitter.
- **Phrase:** This person is just a friend.
- **Translation:** Whenever I get bored, this person is there for me. You might be replaced by them if you leave me.

Complaining about my sneaky behavior with the person will make you look like the overly controlling and jealous one.

- **Phrase:** You're so jealous and insecure.
- **Translation:** I love how you compete for my attention. I feel so powerful and desirable when you get riled up when you see me flirt with others. Making you feel insecure is entertaining, and the less you get diminished, the lesser the chance of you escaping my grasp.
- **Phrases:** You have trust issues.
- **Translation:** I know I am not trustworthy, and I have proven this time and time again. Your intuition is right, but I will never admit it. The only escape plan that can work is to trust yourself and run in the opposite direction, but it won't be fun for me. So, I will use my words to make you feel confused.
- **Phrase:** It's not all about you.
- **Translation:** It is always about me! Your attention should be focused on meeting my needs, and I will make sure that my narcissism is projected to you. I will make sure you feel ashamed for caring for yourself and make sure you don't fulfill your personal needs. Remember, my needs are the only ones that matter.

- **Phrase:** No one would believe you.
- **Translation:** I have made you isolate yourself from others to the point that you no longer have a support system. I have already sullied your name to other people, so they won't suspect that I am lying. People will not believe you because I already painted myself as an amazing person. However, your friends and loved ones might still believe you, and I don't want to risk being caught. So, I make you feel left alone and alienated in order to protect my image. That's my best bet at convincing you to remain silent and not to speak the truth about who I am.
- **Phrase:** You are completely wrong.
- **Translation:** I don't want to listen to what you have to say or whether it is valid. I don't care because it's too much work for me to listen to you.
- **Phrase:** I never said that.
- **Translation:** I may have said that, but I hate how it makes me sound. If I stonewall you this way, you will probably get confused or back off.
- **Phrase:** I think of you as an equal.
- **Translation:** I am telling you this so you will believe that and not see how little I

> think of you. I will be able to manipulate
> you more when you believe this.

Knowing the true meaning behind the words of a narcissist may trigger feelings of anger, grief, relief, freedom, sadness, shock, among others. In the words of the feminist pioneer, Gloria Steinem,

Translating the words of a narcissist who uses gaslighting as a tool for abuse is important because they live a backward life, and you need to figure out their tactic to set yourself free. They always try to be the best in whatever they do to avoid appearing flawed. They act all-powerful to avoid looking weak and always make sure that they avoid appearing ignorant. What they say reflects this endless shell game.

If you are having difficulty translating the narcissist words literally, then you may have stressed and exhausted yourself in the process of making sense out of the words. Even if you try to change your behavior in response to the narcissist's criticisms, the criticism will still continue; because the moment you feel confident is the moment they lose control over you.

To set yourself free from the web of narcissism, you need to pay attention to the actual figure of a narcissist and see them for who they truly are.

FIVE

What Happens to Your Mind?

A s stated earlier, gaslighting has a deep impact on the person who is being abused. As a result of gaslighting, the most affected part is the human mind. The effect of gaslighting takes place gradually, which tends to damage the mind and personality of a person. The process of gaslighting is often slow, and the victim is mostly unaware that they are being gaslighted. They don't realize that their confidence and self-esteem is being chipped away bit by bit. In most cases, the victim may come to believe that they deserve all the abuse that they are getting.

Gaslighting is not just any kind of mind game; it is a very twisted form of abuse where the abuser manipulates their victim's minds with a series of catastrophic effects on the psychological health of the victim. The abuser, in some cases, will employ the victim's confusion and shame to manipulate them into cutting ties or ending relationships with friends, family members, and other people they care about. The abuser takes advantage of their fear to isolate them from others and make the victim totally dependent on the abuser.

Some abusers don't realize that their actions have a miserable effect on their victims until a long time has passed. Meanwhile, this may cause their victims to develop several mental health concerns without the abuser knowing how much damage they are causing to other people. The effect of gaslighting is not just limited to the mind of the victims. The effects spread to their colleagues, friends, and other loved ones of the victim, especially when the victim enters a gaslighting loop, which is a state wherein the victim becomes dependent on the abuser even when they know that they are emotionally abused. They continue to enjoy being with the gaslighter and allow themselves to be manipulated. This process slowly becomes poisonous to the victim's state of mind and the people previously close to the victim of gaslighting.

Over time, the victim of gaslighting may realize that they are not as lively and cheerful as they used to be. This feeling can be overwhelming and heart-breaking for the victim, but they still may not have a solution for how to break away from their abuser. They will continue to feel attached to the gaslighter and will long to be with their abuser. Why? Because they find the gaslighter to be charming. The victim has been manipulated into being dependent and submissive without the power to fight back or resist. The victim will get so used to compromise and forget their experiences. Generally, they don't listen to their inner voice.

Their mind wants to get rid of any poisonous situation they've been through, but they are unable to push themselves to make a decision. Even after realizing that they are being gaslighted, the victim can't trust their own reality or take charge of themselves. And this situation is no less painful or disturbing to those close to the victim because they cannot figure out what is precisely wrong with the person who is being gaslighted, even when they know something is "off" or "strange" about them.

Gaslighting is a mind game that is played between two people, where one is the abuser, and the other is the victim, and the whole process will go largely unnoticed by the victim and those around them. Still, it will keep affecting the mind of the victim, damaging their ability to make proper judgments, breaking down their self-confidence, as well as silently whittling down the mental health of the victim.

The fact is that a gaslighter will have a strong grip on their victim's mind. They can silently control their target with their mind games and keep them in a compliant state. As the victim's mind suffers continuous abuse, their personality will gradually be chipped away bit by bit until little or nothing of their former self is left. All that will be found in their mind will be streams of doubt, low self-esteem, and a total lack of self-confidence. The mind of the gaslighting victim will slowly wear down until they cease to be the person they were before the abuse began.

We will discuss some of the symptoms that describe what happens to the minds of victims of gaslighting below.

Inimical Effects of Gaslighting on The Mind

Loss of self-esteem: a person who is gaslighted by an abuser does not have a high level of self-esteem. When a person has low self-esteem, the basic thing they lack is self- confidence. They can usually be found in situations in which they question their abilities to do something, and they do not believe in themselves at all. A victim of gaslighting will continuously feel bad about themselves and do not know how to respond or reciprocate someone's love and affection. When a victim of gaslighting start to suffer the effect of low self-esteem, they will begin to feel incompetent, awkward, and feel they can't be loved by someone else. Gaslighting affects the minds of abuse victims in such a way that their reality and self-belief gets damaged.

Victims of gaslighting with low self-esteem become overly sensitive and desperate for validation.

They tend to believe that they cannot be right about anything and believe that every task they are asked to perform with others or in a group will go wrong because of them. The gaslighter influences the mind of their victims in a way that their victims develop a deep fear of rejection. They fear that they will lose some of the relationships they possess if they do something wrong. That's why they end up staying quiet and not doing anything about it. All these symptoms arise as a result of low self-esteem, which is a mental health problem for people who are often emotionally abused by the people they know and love the most.

Lack of confidence: victims of gaslighting are often reported to have low confidence in themselves. They find themselves unable to communicate properly with other people and find it even more difficult to correct other matters that they find wrong in their lives. They lack the confidence that their opinions will be taken seriously or that their decisions are correct. Hence, they remain in doubt and feel they will always be wrong. Abuse victims who lack confidence also feel that nothing can go right with them and their actions. They believe that they are a disappointment to others and tend to make other people feel sorry for them. Individuals who face gaslighting feel that they should not do anything and should remain in the condition they're in without making any effort to grow and to have success. If they believe they cannot succeed in any matter of their life, why should they try to better themselves? This perception is what their mind starts to believe after they get manipulated by someone.

Another aspect of low confidence that victims of gaslighting often feel is the fear of incorrect judgments they could make. These people fear to make decisions in their life, even on small matters, because they doubt their own judgments. They don't find themselves eligible or sensible enough to make decisions and think all their decisions are wrong and would lead them towards failure. So, they decide to hand over the right of judgments and decisions to other people around them, some of whom can also be the gaslighters who are the reason for the victim's fear and low confidence.

Isolation: Victims of emotional and psychological abuse often want to isolate themselves from everything and everyone in their life. They start to feel alone and think that no one is there for them. Also, they start to believe that they are not worthy enough to be with someone. They think that everyone hates them and that no one wants to be in their company. All of these mind games that run in their mind are due to the abuser who tends to make them believe that no one is loyal to the victim, and they should not believe anyone. Gaslighters convince their victims that everyone is against them, and they should isolate themselves from the people around them—excluding the gaslighter, of course. The gaslighter makes their victim believe that they are a burden which no one wants to own. Because of all these words and acknowledgments from the gaslighter, the victim decides to isolate themselves so that they do not have to face others.

Emotional shutdown: emotional shutdown is a condition that is faced by a gaslighting victim in which they stop outwardly expressing their emotions. They fear that they will be marked as an oversensitive person. This is why they choose to hide their feelings and emotions and why they are reluctant to share their feelings with others. Victims of gaslighting do not want anyone to know what they are going through or what they tend to feel about any particular thing; they try to avoid being labeled as oversensitive or over-reactive. This is how they go through emotional shutdown in which they choose to shut their mouth and hide their emotions. In such a condition, the victim fears that their emotions are not valid at all. They think that if they try to express their feelings or emotions, they will end up facing other forms of abuse or words like, "this person is too sensitive," or "they don't know how to express themselves." These types of comments from gaslighters make them doubt their own emotions, and they start to take them lightly just to prove that they are not overly sensitive.

Anxiety and depression: when a gaslighting victim remains in a constant state where they doubt themselves, their abilities, and emotions, they start to fall into a mental state known as anxiety. This condition refers to the feeling of the victim in which they feel useless and not able to do anything with their own life. This is an alarming condition for an abuse victim, which then leads to depression. A person with anxiety also feels that they cannot make any sort of decision for themselves and faces problems in this regard, whereas depression is a condition that occurs in a victim of gaslighting when they feel unworthy and out of place. This means that the victim goes into a condition that makes them mentally ill. They feel that they are not worth anything and should not be part of the place they currently belong to.

PTSD (Post Traumatic Stress Disorder): this condition is among the types of mental illness which are caused after a person is gaslighted. In this condition, the victim finds it too difficult to recover from their past experiences and their feelings associated with those incidents. This is an extreme reaction to the trauma and suffering the victim has gone through in the past. This disorder affects the person in a way that changes how the person used to talk, react, think, perceive, feel, and behave. PTSD also causes extreme distress to the victim's mental health, and they undergo a personality change, including the ability for their mind to function properly. This condition can be triggered in a victim of gaslighting, especially if they suffer from extreme gaslighting from an abuser.

Codependency: this is a mental state in which the victim tends to sacrifice their personal need and desires for the happiness and pleasure of other people. They give up on their personal needs in order to help and save others. Such people do not have self-importance at all. This mental condition usually occurs between life partners where one person suffers from having a one-sided relationship, and there is no effort from the other side. The person who is a victim of gaslighting relies on the other person (the gaslighter) for all of their needs, especially those related to their self-esteem and emotional needs. This condition is only painful for the victim, while other people in the relationship get a license to remain irresponsible, addictive, and go about with their unloving behavior. The victim going through this mental condition doesn't want to leave the relationship, but at the same time, they realize that they do not have any free will or choice over their life. They become used to surrendering themselves to the will of another person.

Trust issues: Issues related to trust among relationships may occur as a result of gaslighting. The victim goes through a condition where they find themselves unable to trust anyone. They feel this way because they have had their feelings and trust devastated by many gaslighters already. Such victims will begin to see every other person as a gaslighter and fear that everyone will manipulate them and play with their feelings. They refuse to get close to other people, even shutting out people who could potentially help them through this troubling time in their life. This type of mental condition leads them to ruin healthy relationships and shut out the people they previously trusted. And because they cannot trust anyone anymore, the victim does not care who they are losing.

Lack of focus and productivity: Victims of gaslighting are usually ineffective and inefficient in their tasks. To be able to carry out or complete any task, your mind needs to be active and in the right place. If a person is not mentally active or available, they cannot contribute to their major life problems and tasks. Victims of gaslighting are the least mentally present and find it difficult to focus on their jobs, ambitions, or simple self-care activities. They get distracted easily and cannot show the productivity they should show.

Submissiveness: This phase shows itself in victims of gaslighting when they don't believe in themselves. These victims want to live based on the choices and opinions of other people. In such cases, the victims will want to get a confirmation for everything they need to do in their own life. The gaslighter has devalued the victim in their own eyes that now they want to see themselves from the eyes of other people. They ask for praise from other people. In fact, they need confirmation from other people in every aspect of their life. They seek the validation of others for their actions, completion of daily tasks, and much more. They try to keep such people close who can praise and please them in every aspect of their life. This type of attitude from victims of gaslighting makes them more open to being abused and get mentally tortured because people find it easier to gaslight them and manipulate their minds according to their will.

Being gaslighted is such torture that has very strong and lasting effects on the victim's mind.

.

SIX

What Happens to Your Body?

Although gaslighting is mostly a mental form of abuse and manipulation, its effects have been known to spill over into the physical self. As we learned from the last chapter, there is a myriad of mental issues that can arise from one being gaslit. This can lead to excessive amounts of stress, which in turn translates to a wide variety of ailments on your body. The effects include but aren't limited to the few we are going to explore in-depth in this chapter.

Insomnia

Insomnia is defined as a sleeping disorder where one has trouble falling or staying asleep. It can be either acute (that is, it can be short-term, lasting anywhere from one night to a few weeks) or chronic (meaning long-term, happening at least three nights a week for three months).

There are two distinct types of insomnia:

- **Primary Insomnia:** Where one's lack of sleep isn't linked to any health condition or current problem.
- **Secondary Insomnia:** Where the root cause of one being unable to sleep can be linked back to a health condition. A few common examples include asthma, depression, cancer, and anxiety.

Mental health issues like depression and anxiety are the most common causes of secondary insomnia, and both are major side effects of gaslighting—which is unsurprising. After all, the nagging thought that you are slowly losing your mind is guaranteed to keep you up at night. How can you sleep if you fear that you are losing touch with reality? How can you sleep when a person you love is out to disrupt your life and make you question your every sense?

Unlike other illnesses whereby the symptoms are indicative of a far more sinister root cause, the opposite is often true of insomnia.

The symptoms of insomnia include fatigue, sleepiness, grumpiness, and problems with concentration or memory. These symptoms go further beyond the surface problems they cause. These symptoms can decrease your interaction with other people in your social circle since you are always tired. The forgetfulness that can arise from insomnia can also further support your abuser's point that you forget details. Now, when you truly forget details of conversations or remember things wrong, your mind tells you, "You see? They were right. You do forget things." This new realization will make you rely more on your abuser, leaving you vulnerable to more abuse.

This doesn't begin to cover the safety risks posed by going through the day only half awake and being expected to complete basic tasks like driving and operating machinery, which can have tragic consequences. Insomnia can lead to poor performance at school and/or work. In class, you are not fully alert to pick up lessons. In the workplace, you are sluggish, and you miss deadlines. Missed deadlines plus sluggishness equals to stagnancy at work.

Our brains and bodies need sleep so they can repair themselves, and it is also crucial for learning and storing memories. Continued insomnia can lead to higher blood pressure, trouble focusing, and obesity, among a slew of other health problems.

Chronic Pain

Pain can be said to be the body's early warning system; it is the body's way of letting you know that something is wrong.

Normal pain has a shelf life—as soon as the injury heals, you stop hurting. That is not the case with chronic pain. For chronic pain, your body keeps hurting for months and even years after the initial injury. It can be defined as any pain that lasts for three to six months or more and can have serious effects on your day-to-day life.

Chronic pain can occur continually throughout the day. At other times, it can come and go, and its intensity varies wildly from mild discomfort to severe unimaginable pain. It occurs as a dull ache, soreness, stiffness, a throbbing pain, a burning sensation, muscle tension, back pains, migraines, and chest pains.

Its symptoms can also include a loss of appetite, trouble sleeping, mood changes, a lack of energy, and general overall weakness and apathy.

The link between pain and a person's emotions can create a feedback loop, and when you're depressed, you're more likely to feel pain and vice versa, which is why it is common practice in the health and wellness industry to treat chronic pain with antidepressants. So, do you now see how gaslighting can cause you chronic pain? When you are depressed continually, it can lead to pain, which can lead to difficulty in other aspects of your life.

Self-Harm, Suicide

Depression and a lack of self-worth brought about by years of being gaslighted have been known to take a huge toll on an individual. It is no surprise then that a majority of gaslighting victims have admitted to considering the option of ending their own lives or seeking dangerous outlets for their emotions as they feel that they are their own worst enemies, which is far from true.

Extreme gaslighting can cause you to question your very existence. What's worse is that the person who is supposed to help you out of this mess is the person responsible for your problems. It becomes even worse when you remember how sweet that person used to be. You will begin to wonder what happened. Your gaslighter will keep giving you the impression that you caused the change in their attitude, making it even worse for you.

Some universal symptoms for major depression, if left unchecked, could lead to self-harm or suicide. These symptoms include:

- A persistent sad or empty mood
- Feeling hopeless, helpless, worthless, pessimistic and/or guilty
- Irritability, increased crying, anxiety, or panic attacks

- Thoughts of suicide, including suicide plans and/or attempts
- Persistent physical symptoms or pains that don't respond to medical treatment
- Disturbances in eating and sleeping patterns
- Fatigue or loss of interest in ordinary activities
- Increasing the use of alcohol or drugs
- Displaying extreme mood swings
- Talking about feeling trapped and wanting to die

These are common symptoms of mental health issues caused by gaslighting. Some victims might even seek relief in substance abuse. The bottom line is that emotional pain can be more destabilizing than physical pain.

Thankfully, suicide is preventable. It is a complex public health issue that requires cooperation among family members, individuals, health care providers, and the community at large. If we all work together, we can increase public awareness of this public health issue and get people the help and support they need.

Since you are reading this, I hope that you will learn to work the effects of gaslighting and live your best life. If you've ever considered suicide due to abuse before, I will suggest that in addition to reading this book, consider visiting a therapist who will recommend some meditation for you to help you bounce back on your feet.

Eating Disorders

The term, "To eat one's feelings," is a universal one in the English-speaking world for a reason. Since the dawn of time, eating has always been a pleasure for mankind, and for most people, it serves as a coping mechanism. Binge-eating is a way to distract us from the death of a beloved family pet, losing a job, or going through a divorce or a particularly difficult breakup.

There is no denying that food can be comforting, which is probably why we have certain foods that are referred to as comfort food. The reason food is so comforting is because trauma causes an increase in anxiety and frustration and eating serves to trigger a physiological release and a neurochemical surge that serves to alter the mood and distract one from their trauma.

Now, imagine being in a relationship with the source of your trauma, getting sucked into a never-ending cycle of abuse, and then eating your feelings to try and cope. With time, the eating that initially provided an escape, protection, and calm in your life spirals out of control. You indulge in emotional eating, which is characterized by the indiscriminate consumption of anything that comes your way. This continued assault on the body will eventually destroy one's health, leading to obesity and related health issues and have been known to lead to death.

Body Dysmorphia

Body dysmorphia sometimes referred to as dysmorphophobia, is a mental illness wherein an individual obsessively fixates on some aspect of their own body or appearance and perceives it to be defective or severely flawed. As a result, they become so embarrassed, ashamed, and anxious about their appearance that they go to extraordinary lengths and take exceptional measures to hide or fix this supposed flaw/defect that appears minor or can't be seen by others. It is a figment of one's imagination, and even if it is real, its importance is severely exaggerated. This may cause you to avoid a multitude of social situations, thoughts about this perceived flaw may occupy you for several hours a day, causing significant distress, impacting your ability to function and go about your normal daily lives.

Body dysmorphia is a common effect of gaslighting, as one of the techniques favored by gaslighters is constantly harping on an imagined or slight flaw that they know the victim is insecure about. They do this to keep their victim unsure and to make them perpetually uneasy in their skin and constantly question themselves, therefore seeking the gaslighter's validation to make them feel better.

The abuser might never even make remarks on your appearance (although they can as well), but the victim needs to be attractive to them, and "worthy" of them. These irrational—and often impossible—standards can lead to eating disorders such as anorexia or bulimia. In some cases, the obsession will cause the victim to seek out a string of cosmetic surgeries to try to "fix" the perceived flaw. This may lead to a feeling of temporary satisfaction or a reduction in their distress, but more often than not, the anxiety returns and the search for other ways to fix this perceived "flaw" resumes.

Unhealthy Outlets for Emotion

Skin Picking. Skin picking disorder also referred to as Dermatillomania or Excoriation disorder, is believed to affect as many as 1 in every 20 people. It is among a subsection of behaviors known as body-focused repetitive behaviors. It's a compulsive habit associated with anxiety—quite similar to OCD (Obsessive Compulsive Disorder)—in which the sufferer repeatedly scratches, picks, rubs, or digs at their skin with fingernails or tools like tweezers. This compulsive behavior can potentially cause damage resulting in bleeding, wounds, sores, and scarring.

The impacts can be psychological as well. After

all, if we have a problem with our skin, it makes us feel low and reluctant to engage with the world until the "flaw" is fixed. At extreme levels, sufferers can end up needing plastic surgery or can contract secondary infections like Necrotizing Fasciitis, more commonly known as flesh-eating disease.

How can gaslighting cause this? Never underestimate anything that can affect your mental wellness. This is why there is so much awareness of gaslighting. People are waking up to the health impacts that a gaslighter can inflict on their victims.

Obsession. Obsessions refer to periods where we find ourselves utterly fascinated with a thought or an idea that we can't seem to shake. Instead, these thoughts continually circulate around and around in our minds. Obsessions turn into anxious obsessions when the content of the thought plaguing the sufferer is of particular personal dread. The thoughts can either be plausible or implausible. An example of a plausible anxious obsession would be of a loved one dying or a relationship failing, whereas an example of an implausible obsession would be a dread of one getting abducted by aliens.

Equally distressing is when the obsessive thoughts seem to run contrary to one's moral code. An example is when a happily married person is having anxious, obsessive thoughts about leaving their spouse. Here the person becomes quite distressed about the seemingly "unnatural." Seen in this light, one could say that anxious obsessions are merely distressing, long, and repetitive versions of atypical anxious thoughts. It is the relentlessness that can make it feel unmanageable.

Gaslighting can make you depressed because you believe that nobody will want to be around you if they fear that they are losing touch with reality. Nobody will be happy if they have to rely on somebody to think for them, listen for them, see for them, and feel for them.

Heart Disease

Emotional trauma, such as repeated mental abuse, can increase the risk of a heart attack. Psychological disorders and psychological stressors have been proven to be linked to various heart problems. People who suffer from depression are more at risk of suffering from heart attacks. They are more likely to develop conditions that increase heart risks like high blood pressure, obesity, and an irregular heart rate.

People who suffer from chronic anxiety (like those being gaslighted) are twice as likely to suffer atrial fibrillation and sudden death brought on by their high blood pressure and stuttering heart rate. Intense bouts of emotion have been known to bring about long-lasting heart damage. What stress hormones do today can have a quite substantial impact on how healthy our cardiovascular system will be a couple of decades from now.

Real-time physical effects have been known to even correlate with acute emotional states. This phenomenon is known as Takotsubo Cardiomyopathy —also known as stress cardiomyopathy or broken heart syndrome. It is more prevalent in women than men and, compared with people who had experienced a "typical" heart attack, patients with Takotsubo cardiomyopathy are almost twice as likely to have a neurological ailment as an adjacent component.

Acid Reflux

Gastroesophageal reflux (commonly referred to as Heartburn) or acid reflux is a painful burning feeling in your chest or your throat, it is caused when the esophagus (the tube responsible for shuttling food to your stomach from your mouth) relaxes too much, and stomach acid comes back up into your esophagus. Although anxiety won't cause GERD (Gastroesophageal Reflux Disease), it can cause heartburn and exacerbate GERD symptoms, making them much worse.

A person can have both GERD- related heartburn and anxiety-related heartburn. For such a person, treating with acid-suppressing medication does not alleviate the problem. And in some cases, acid reflux acts up at the worst possible times—say before a job interview, in the middle of a fight or before a big presentation. This could indicate that it isn't GERD-related heartburn, but rather anxiety-related heartburn, and this type of acid reflux should be treated accordingly.

Ulcers

A stress-induced ulcer is a fairly common acute erosive or ulcerative lesion of the stomach and duodenum that occurs in tandem with and response to stressful physical or mental situations. An ulcer occurs when tissue in a section of the mouth, stomach, or esophagus becomes damaged. The section becomes inflamed and irritated and creates a hole or a sore.

An untreated ulcer may, in some cases, cause the following acute symptoms:

- Loss of appetite and weight loss
- Difficulty Breathing
- Internal bleeding
- Vomiting
- Nausea
- Lightheadedness

Rashes

The growth of rashes on the skin is a common physical symptom of stress and anxiety. In isolation, mild forms of stress have a small effect on the body. However, frequent exposure to stress can trigger quite a few adverse side effects.

Stress causes several hormonal or chemical changes in the body that makes skin more reactive and sensitive and can go as far as making it harder for skin problems to heal. These changes can make the blood vessels expand and leak, causing red swollen patches of skin and can also cause the body to produce more hormones like cortisol—whose presence signals glands in your skin to make more oil—and oily skin is more prone to acne and other numerous skin problems.

Luckily, a stress-induced rash is rarely a cause for concern, and it can be treated at home, although it bears mentioning that stress can exacerbate pre-existing skin conditions like psoriasis, rosacea, or eczema. Stress rashes often manifest in the form of hives (also called wheals or welts), which unfortunately can appear anywhere on the body. Areas affected by hives traditionally present as generally red-colored spots, raised and/or swollen skin. The areas affected by these blotchy nuisances can be as tiny as a pencil tip or as big as a dinner plate. The patches may even connect to form even larger blotches covering large areas of the skin.

Areas affected by hives can feel itchy. In some cases, they might cause a slight tingling or a burning sensation when touched. When stressed, it isn't uncommon to experience a flare-up connected to a pre-existing skin condition. The reason is that your body releases extra chemicals such as neuropeptides and neurotransmitters when one is stressed. These chemicals then change how your body responds to a plethora of functions. Changes in your body's reactions can then cause inflammation, sensitivity, and other skin discomforts.

In conclusion, gaslighting should not be taken lightly because it not only affects your mind; it also affects your physical body, and these physical effects can be damaging to your health in the long run.

SEVEN

Can You Avoid Being Gaslighted?

W e've learned all about gaslighters and how they operate. We've also seen the undesirable physical and mental effects gaslighting can have on us. The big question now is, "Can gaslighting be avoided? And if so, how?" I will give a thorough answer to this burning question so that you can protect yourself from gaslighters going forward.

First of all, yes, gaslighting can be avoided. Make no mistake, it will not always be easy, but the truth is that you can avoid being gaslighted. I say it is not easy because if you fail to recognize gaslighting for what it is, you won't be able to avoid it. Thankfully, awareness is the first step to protect yourself.

Trust Your Gut

The subject of gaslighting can be a tricky one, especially when emotion is involved. Gaslighters are so good at their craft of manipulation that it could take a long time for you to notice the patterns. They will keep telling you that they are actually looking out for you, but by reading this book, I know you now know how to identify if you are being gaslighted. The first step to avoiding it is by identifying it. If your gut tells you that something is off, you should believe it. Trust your instinct on this, because if your partner or whoever gives you room to think that you are being gaslighted, then you probably are. But if you are still not sure, try discussing it with a trusted friend, relative, or even a therapist. However, the easiest way to check is to look inwards and see if you are beginning to doubt yourself due to your relationship with somebody.

First Thing First, Talk Things Over

Let's say you have confirmed that you are being gaslighted by someone. The first thing you should do is talk it over with whoever is involved. Sometimes, your partner can be gaslighting you unintentionally. In this case, you must assess the situation and see if they are doing it in a bid to control you or if they are doing it because they are struggling with the idea of not being in control. Either way, it still hurts.

If the gaslighter is not doing it intentionally, there just might be a little beam of hope. The best way to proceed is to talk with them. This might be difficult, but it is worth a try. You can start by letting your partner know that they've been dismissing your feelings lately and let them know how it makes you feel. If the gaslighter responds favorably, and it becomes clear that they are not intentionally trying to control you, you both can look for a better way to communicate and relate.

However, if the gaslighter is doing it intentionally, you can still try to talk about it. The best time to bring this up is when the atmosphere is friendly or when you both are in a good mood. This is important because if you bring it up in the middle of an argument, your gaslighter might misunderstand it for an attack, and that wouldn't go over well. Also, before talking about it, warn the gaslighter by telling them that you've noticed something lately. Let them know that it bothers you and that you would like to talk about it.

Then, proceed forward with the conversation in the friendliest manner you can. The best way will be to negotiate around the topic and to not be blunt about it. If you decide to be blunt, the gaslighter might get defensive and dismiss your thoughts once again. But if you proceed in a friendly manner and they don't get defensive, it is time to let them know that you want to hear their side of the situation and where they are coming from. Let them know that you will understand if there is something they've been going through lately and if they would want to share their feelings with you. If they come up plain and you see reasons with them, let them know that you really want to keep the relationship going, but that you want to have a voice too and not be always dismissed.

Seek External Help Together

This applies to people who are being gaslighted by their partners. If you still want to try to repair the relationship rather than just giving up, you can opt to see a therapist together—if your partner is compliant, that is. Sometimes it can be difficult for both of you to see each other's perspective. A little help from a therapist could help your partner see your plight and will help you to see theirs. And if in truth, you are just being too sensitive, which is very unlikely, the therapist will be in a better position to tell you so because they will be unbiased in their judgment.

Also, a counselor might help you both have key conversations that are necessary. They will just listen and help channel the conversation to pressing issues that you and your partner might be oblivious of.

But if your gaslighter is intentionally trying to abuse you, seeing a third party together can shut down their abilities because if a third party will call them out on their lies. This third party means that they lose their ability to control you through mind games because now they know that you (as well as an outside party) know their games and tactics. The gaslighter would have to be insane to try the same lies on you again.

If you try all of these and it doesn't yield any results, or if the gaslighter becomes defensive and tries to dismiss what you are saying, it is time to adopt stricter measures that will be discussed below.

First, in order for you to avoid being gaslighted, you have to know the ways the gaslighter will try to gaslight you. We've discussed common gaslighting tactics in chapter 4 of this book. However, let's look at them again briefly so I can show you how you can practically handle these techniques when the gaslighter tries to use them on you.

Withholding: the gaslighter will try to act like they don't understand what you are telling them. They may also refuse to listen to whatever you are saying to them. When you notice this, ensure that you get the abuser to understand you. You can tell them that it seems like they do not understand what you are saying and that you will really appreciate it if they can listen to you and understand what you are saying. It is important to consciously get the abuser to understand you so that when they try to twist something you said, your subconscious mind will make it obvious to you that it is a gaslighting scheme. This time, you are very sure that the gaslighter heard you right the first time.

Countering: a gaslighter may try to get you to doubt your memory so that you will feel you've lost it and depend solely on them. One way you can prevent this is by keeping a journal. Write down key events in your life and update it regularly. If the gaslighter comes at you and tries to make it seem like you are losing touch with reality, you can simply refer to your journal and reassure yourself that your memory is fine. When you realize that your version of the past even is correct, you will see the abuser for who they are, and you will begin to trust your sanity again.

Sometimes, a gaslighter might promise to reward you with something when you do something for them. When you do your part, and it is their turn to keep to their words, they will turn things around and make you doubt your memory. But since you already know them for who they are, you will be cautious with them, and that means recording those promises in a journal so you can pull it up and remind them of it later.

Blocking and diverting: in my years of counseling abuse victims, I have identified this tactic as something that gaslighters like to use very often. The gaslighter will always try to make conversations very unbearable for your sanity. They will attempt to block and divert any talk that can reaffirm your sanity. They will try to distort information so that you begin to doubt your hearing and reasoning. The way to prevent this is to reach within and tell yourself that you hear right and that there is nothing wrong with your reasoning. You can also record the conversations and have a third party you trust to listen to it. Let them assess it and see if their assessment of the situation is any different from yours.

Trivializing: your abuser will try to belittle your thoughts and emotions, usually by claiming or implying that you are too sensitive and have no reason to feel the way you feel. In this case, if you are not sure whether you are truly overreacting or not, you can confide in a trusted person and tell them all about it. Then, ask them if they honestly think that you are overreacting.

Forgetting and denial: in their attempt to manipulate you, the abuser will also try to deny occurrences of the past. To stop these denials, use journaling to keep yourself from questioning your memory. As you engage with the gaslighter, record everything that happened, and state how the events made you feel. You can also add when it happened for easy reference. It is important that you record how it made you feel because by doing that, you are validating your emotions, and that can help you resist manipulation. Your journal will also be there to set the records straight whenever you are tempted to question your memory and sanity.

Trust Your Intuition

The gaslighter is only able to sway you when you start distrusting your intuition. There are several techniques, such as mindfulness and meditation, that you can use to always remain in the moment.

Mindfulness will help you make a note of the happenings around you. You will not just be swayed by a gaslighter because you distrust your own intuition. By trusting your intuition, I mean that you must learn how to stand up and defend what your intuition tells you. If and when you stop listening to your voice, then you are gradually submitting to gaslighting. To avoid being gaslighted, you need to fight back by standing up for yourself and your feelings. Also, it will help you to remember what and how you feel.

Victims that have been gaslighted for a long period of time often stop listening to their own voice. After all, what's the point in listening to yourself if you're always being criticized? To reclaim your inner voice, you can start meditating and journaling. When you are aware of your emotions, you will know how to fight back.

How Can You Avoid Being Gaslighted?

Education. The first step to avoiding being gaslighted is education. Being able to spot the tell-tale signs of gaslighting can be a deciding factor in whether or not you'll become a victim. Many people become victims of gaslighting because they do not know how gaslighters operate. They spend most of their time thinking that they are the problem, so the gaslighter just continues abusing them. It is a good thing that you are educating yourself on gaslighting by reading this book. And by now, I believe you know the modus operandi of gaslighters. So, when next you encounter a narcissist or a gaslighter, and they try to pull a fast one on you, quickly remind yourself that you are not the problem—they are the problem.

One trick you can use to remind yourself that the gaslighter is the problem is to understand that they are probably doing it because they are trying to remedy their low self-esteem, or perhaps it is because they're trying to regain control of their own lives. Once you convince yourself that they are acting the way they do because of their personal battles, you will learn to consider their treatments lightly, and this means more control for you. Now that you are not taking them as seriously, you are regaining the power you were being denied in the relationship.

The ability to understand that they are the problem and not you will help you regain control of your life and position. It will also be easier to not take what they say personally, thus thwarting their plans and goals to manipulate you.

Get outside advice. Gaslighters aim to have you not trust your own mind. If you are unable to clearly judge your position, feelings, or reasoning, get someone you trust to help you assess the situation. This step is important early on, as a gaslighter might try to make you distrust those people. But you must learn to get outside advice because if you only listen to your gaslighter, they will confuse you even further. The way out is meant to help you keep your external relationships as strong as possible. It is even possible for your friends and families to notice something off and help you so that you don't get swallowed up by the abuse.

In terms of your external relationships, if you break off from a gaslighter in the process of avoiding gaslighting, you may need a sturdy support system (outside relationships); this is especially crucial if the gaslighter is your partner. If you do not have this support system in place, the gaslighter might maneuver their way back into your life.

Remove yourself from the situation. At work, if you are unable to change positions or companies, you can have HR assess the situation and help you work out a way in which you will not have to work with the gaslighter. This may lead to the abuser switching to another target if they find a suitable one. Spreading information on gaslighting around can be helpful to others as well.

In the family, it may be more difficult. You can move (even to a different city) if you have the ability to do so. Try to cut off all contact with the gaslighter.

In relationships, it's vital to recognize the symptoms early on. Otherwise, you may get pulled into the abuser's scheme. End a relationship with a gaslighter as soon as possible.

Sometimes, it might not be easy for you to just walk out on the abuser like when they are a co-worker, and you cannot easily change jobs. In such cases, you can disarm your abuser using techniques I will discuss with you in the next chapter.

Change your Perspective

Shift your perspective from being a victim to being a warrior, winner, or whatever word feels the most empowering to you. You don't have to remain a victim for the rest of your life, and by reclaiming your personal power, you'll also be able to help others in similar circumstances.

Ignore Motives

Most gaslighters have a motive for their gaslighting, and more often than not, it is to control you. There could be other reasons like we saw in the film *Gaslight* where Gregory's motive was to steal Paula's inheritance. But you must ignore the motives. If you don't, you will be further trapping yourself because it will never be apparent, and it will increase your confusion and self-doubt.

Using Cognitive Behavioral Therapy to Avoid Gaslighting

As you already know, gaslighting thrives on your perception of yourself. While the methods and steps we've discussed so far can help you avoid gaslighting, it may be difficult for you alone to handle, especially if the gaslighter has firmly wrapped their hands around your mind. Cognitive-behavioral therapy (CBT) is a type of therapy that is concerned with your perception of yourself. It looks at the impact of your thoughts on your behavior. It is also effective for other mental health issues such as anxiety and depression.

For us to see just how CBT can help you avoid gaslighting, let's look at the ABC's of gaslighting. The ABC's stand for Activating, Belief, and Consequences. Activating is the issue that triggers the belief that brings about the consequences. In the case of gaslighting, the gaslighter's attitude towards you is the activating. This activating is not really the cause of your trauma; it is the thought or interpretation you give to it that brings about the consequences, which is the trauma. So, if you interpret the gaslighter's actions to mean that your instincts are not correct and you are insane, then the trauma sets in. But if you refuse to interpret it that way, then you will save yourself from the impending trauma. CBT says that if you allow yourself to accommodate negative thoughts always, then it will weigh you down. That is why you can use CBT to not feel what the gaslighter wants you to feel.

Another reason why CBT can help you avoid gaslighting is that a therapist uses structured sessions to get you to become aware of the lies and deceit around you. If you become more aware of the situation around you, then it is very unlikely that you will allow it to get to you.

CBT is a therapy that will require a therapist to carry out effectively. So, you might need to contact a therapist to help you avoid becoming a gaslighting victim or falling back into old habits.

EIGHT

Moving Forward - Disarming

S ometimes, you cannot just pick up your things and walk out on a gaslighter. They may be your benefactor, or you may be married to them and have children with them—and now you are scared of having your kids go through the trauma of a parent's divorce. It could also be that you are gainfully employed somewhere, and your gaslighting is of the workplace type. Some other times, you cannot simply walk away because you love the gaslighter so much, and you believe that they can change. There are several scenarios that might make it difficult to just break free from a gaslighter. In that case, the best option available to you is to disarm the gaslighter. This chapter will explain some techniques of the first stage of fighting back: disarming the gaslighter, removing their tools, and putting up the first line of defense.

If you have to be in contact with a gaslighter, it's important to minimize the damage they can do to you and even avoid that damage completely.

Keep a Log of Events and Conversations

Having written, material evidence of what happened can help take away some power from the gaslighter. They will try to deny it all anyway, but if you make it a practice, they may realize that it will be harder to get to you

Since gaslighters thrive on denying and lying, having a witness to your conversations with them can also be helpful. An outsider (a co-worker, another family member, etc.) can later vouch for one of you. If the gaslighter denies and lies, you will have someone to validate your claims and to keep you grounded. Validating your claim might be all you need to not doubt your reasoning. Since the gaslighter is out to make you believe that you imagine things, having someone else believe your version/reality will also make it harder for the gaslighter to convince you that you imagine things.

It will be harder in relationships, as a lot of the gaslighting happens in private. In that case, there might not be a third party to serve as a witness when there is a denial.

Get Back in Touch with Your Intuition and Feelings

To disarm a gaslighter, you need to stand up for your emotions and yourself. But you need to first remember what and how you feel. Victims that have suffered from prolonged gaslighting often stop listening to their own voice since they're always criticized. Meditation, journaling, and other mindful activities can help you get back to having your own thoughts and being certain of them

Avoid Direct Confrontation

One of the ways in which the gaslighter will react is blame-shifting. Because they're often inclined to project, they may try to turn the table and cast the same accusation on you if you accuse them of gaslighting; or they may resort to personal attacks.

Name What's Happening

Giving the issue a name makes it more "tangible" and manageable. Make sure you call what's happening "gaslighting", at least to yourself. It can be helpful to also call it out loud to others. When you identify what is going on, you become aware of the pattern of undermining behavior. So when the gaslighter uses their tactics on you, you can immediately recognize it for what it is and shrug it off immediately.

Rebuild Your Self-Esteem

Work on rebuilding your self-esteem. The gaslighter will try to make it seem like you are an unlovable person, but you mustn't allow that. The opinion of the gaslighter is just one in thousands of people that know you, and I'm sure you have other people around you that love you for who you are. You can easily grow your self-esteem by reminding yourself of the time before you met the gaslighter—when you felt sane, secured, loved, and safe. So, if you don't feel good about yourself now, then it has everything to do with the gaslighter and not with you. If it is difficult for you to recall those good times, maybe due to the level of damage that the gaslighter has done, you may opt to recall your positive memories gradually and write them down in your journal.

Check to See If Your Conversations are Power Struggles

How do you know if it is a power struggle? When you notice that the person you are dealing with is attempting to gain the upper hand and prove that they are right and that you are wrong. If you are not careful, you too will be struggling to get the approval of the gaslighter to get them to see the situation the way you see it; but then we know that is never going to happen.

A power struggle is different from a real conversation. In a real conversation, there is no battle for who is right or wrong. Rather, you and your partner are more concerned with listening to each other's concerns, and your primary concern is to sort things out amicably so that both of you leave the conversation feeling heard. Anything different from this is a power struggle, and you know better than to get into a power struggle with a gaslighter because you will never win. Rather, you will experience the gaslighting effect some more.

Gaslighters thrive more when you engage with them. They want you both to go on with the back and forth conversations about who is right and who is not. Don't give them that chance. Don't engage with them. To them, it is like a game, and they need somebody to play it with. You can stay with them and choose not to play the game. If you do that, you won't be sucked into the manipulation. Instead of going on with the power struggle, recognize it for what it is, and tell the gaslighter that you don't want to proceed with the conversation.

Call Them Out

A confrontation is never an option when disarming a gaslighter because things can go sideways. But you have a better option than confrontation, and it is calling them out. You can let the gaslighter know that you know what they are trying to do to you. Tell them that you are not willing to partake in this sort of relationship and that you want it to stop. This will deflate their ego and disarm them because now they know that you are aware of all their subtle manipulations. It would be stupid of them to try and manipulate you ever again.

Sort Out Truth from Distortion

When you are dealing with a gaslighter, be prepared to hear different versions of any given event, an act that is meant to confuse you. They are masters at this, so they will include some truths in what they say to get you to believe the whole story. But now that you know you are dealing with a gaslighter, you may need to always go the extra mile to find out the truth. Clarify your thinking and sort out the truth from the lies. It is not a difficult thing. You just have to look at the two sides of what they tell you. They will always be the real thing and something else that they want you to believe. For instance, they may tell you that you are overreacting to something that is not worth this amount of attention. But then you know within you that the issue is worth the attention you are giving it. Now you have identified the distortion which is aimed at making you look crazy.

Hold on to What You Know Is True

Gaslighting is characterized by lies, deceits, and manipulation, but you can disarm your gaslighter if you hold on to the things you know are true. No matter what the gaslighter does to make you doubt the obvious things that you know, do not allow yourself to be swayed by them. They will lie to you, distort the meaning of your words, and deny events. All of these are aimed at misdirecting you. But the misdirection can only happen if you allow it. You may have been lied to before, but you can carefully pick out the truths and hold on to them, come rain or come shine. Doing this will eliminate the seeds of self-doubt that the gaslighter is doing everything to plant into you. And when you refuse to permit self-doubt, you are better equipped to see the schemes being plotted by the gaslighter.

Identify the Gaslight Triggers

When you are involved with a gaslighter, there will always be certain things that trigger the gaslighting process. You can take some time and look over all the times your gaslighter has tried to manipulate you and see the main issues that led to it. Once you identify those triggers, you can avoid them altogether, or you avoid talking about those things with them. The triggers may fall into broad categories, which include certain situations, topics, words. Some examples are money, sex, children, cheating, and inheritance, among others. You will have to identify which trigger is used in your dynamic with a gaslighter.

The best way to identify those triggers is to look at the topics you would rather not talk about with your gaslighter because it scares you. If your instinct is avoiding them, then you should make conscious efforts to avoid them altogether.

Focus on the Way You Feel, Not on Whether You are "Right" or "Wrong". When a gaslighter wants to accuse you, they will attach a little truth to their lie and go on to blow it out of proportion. This is done in order to leave you wondering if they are right or wrong. And it can be hard deciding this because there will be some form of truth to it, making it difficult for you to decide if they are right or just manipulating you.

Let me illustrate with an example. Let's say that you and your gaslighting partner attend a party and you meet up with an old friend. Because it's been a while, you get caught up in the moment and spend a good amount of time with your friend. Your partner might conclude that you were flirting and that you did it intentionally to humiliate them. Now, you can't say for sure if that is what it seems like. You may become confused in the moment, but you know deep down that all you did was communicate freely with a long-lost friend.

The best way to proceed in such a case is to check your feelings rather than trying to decide if they are right or wrong. If, by checking your feelings, you discover that you are guilty of what you are being accused of and you feel remorse, you can apologize. But if you feel attacked or bewildered, that means you are being gaslighted, and the best way to proceed is to disengage immediately.

Realize That You Can't Control Their Opinion. Some victims of gaslighting remain victims for so long because they erroneously believe that they can change the opinion of the gaslighter. But we know that this might never happen. Rather than trying to change their opinion, choose freedom instead. Let me give you a scenario. If your partner is doing something that you know for sure is not right (like consuming too much alcohol), and you are busy trying to make them see reasons with you, they may tell you that you are too sensitive, and you might start to consider the possibility of them being right.

So, you see that this situation could have been avoided if you hadn't tried to change their opinion about alcohol. No matter what you tell them about the effects of excessive alcoholism, a gaslighter will always hold on to their opinions on alcoholism. So, if you know that trying to change them will only gaslight you further, then you need to let it be.

Don't Show that You're an Empath

Empaths are more likely to be gaslighted because they are very sensitive to the energy of people around them. Since they care so much about the energy of people around them, they tend to be too self-sacrificing because they just want people to be happy. They are also known as energy sponges because they can soak up whatever energy is thrown their way. Gaslighters and narcissists find empaths to be easy prey, and once they discover that you are one, they hook in and sap out all of that empathy until you become a shadow of your former self.

Being an empath is not your choice, but controlling your empathy is. We live in a cold world where everybody cannot be like you. As an empath, you will find it very hard to believe that somebody will want to hurt you despite your kindness toward them.

If you wish to disarm a gaslighter, you must be resolute with your emotions and never show your weakness as an empath. But if you have tried and you just can't stand up for yourself, then at least realize your weaknesses as an empath and protect yourself at all costs.

Certain empathic attributes that maybe your undoing are:

1. You will struggle to differentiate your emotions from those of your abuser

because you will always want to feel what they feel and look out for them. If you do that, you will be easy prey that will be manipulated with ease.

2. You will lack personal boundaries, and you might not know how to say "no" to outrageous requests from your abuser. Bottom line, you will be a people pleaser, and that can prove to be very deadly for you in the hands of a gaslighter.

The gaslighter will manipulate you with ease because, even when you know that they are manipulating you, you will not speak up because you don't want to hurt their feelings. And if you lack the ability to say "no", you are the perfect prey for all the gaslighting techniques we discussed earlier in this book.

In conclusion, there are subtle ways you can "turn off the gas"; but that's if you decide that you don't want to leave the gaslighter, which might actually be the best option for you.

I hear stories of people advocating that you should give the gaslighter a taste of their own medicine. They say you can get them to be silent when you manipulate them back and shout at them. While that might work temporarily, it is still a dangerous thing to do because they will always come for revenge. And assuming that they don't come for revenge, do you really want to sink down to using a gaslighter's tactics? If you do, you would be reducing yourself to their moral level.

But if you decide that you want to stay and fight, then you can use the tips we've discussed to effectively disarm your gaslighter. Note that disarming them does not mean that you have changed them; it only means that you have figured out how to handle their manipulations.

They won't just accept defeat like that; they will look for newer responses to your disarming tactics, so you must be prepared to evolve as well and never let your guard down. In the next chapter, I will show you ways you can finally break free from a gaslighter if disarming them might not be the best option available to you.

NINE

Moving Forward - Breaking Free

S ometimes, it becomes obvious that you just cannot continue putting up with a gaslighter. You have done all you can to block off their subtle manipulations, but it seems like you are losing yourself at every step along the way. If this is the case, the most reasonable thing for you to do is to break free from the gaslighter completely. Granted, this is much easier said than done. It may be the most difficult thing you will have to do in your relationship. But one thing is certain—it is worth it. I will use this chapter to show you how you can actually remove yourself from that toxic relationship that is threatening your sanity.

People who are in love with a gaslighter are always caught in that nasty web of believing that they can change them. Even though that is possible, it is rare;

and even in those rare cases, you may not be able to reform a gaslighter on your own. They may require a therapist to help them with the bad self-image that is usually the main cause of gaslighting in a person.

So, what can be done to break free from the influence of a gaslighter, especially if they cannot be or don't want to be reformed?

First, you must identify that you are being gaslighted. We've gone through that in earlier chapters of this book, but here is a quick refresher—if your relationship lacks consideration, mutual respect, and trust, that is the first sign. And if you find yourself second-guessing yourself, that is a confirmation that your partner has been toying with your reasoning.

Do not make the mistake of believing that you can easily spot a gaslighter. Many factors can cloud your perception, making it hard for you to realize that the person you love is manipulating you. The first factor is emotions, especially if it is somebody you are romantically involved with. The second is that, unlike physical and verbal abuse that is easier to identify, it is very difficult to identify emotional or psychological abuse because of its subtle nature. If you are waiting for your gaslighter to explode into angry fights, argue violently with you, or throw tantrums, you may have to wait forever because they don't operate in that manner. Your gaslighter might even have you under the erroneous belief that they are doing what they are doing because they love you.

The first step to breaking free from your gaslighter is acknowledging the signs in your relationship.

Breaking Free from Gaslighting in General

The goal is to become free of the influence of the gaslighter altogether. They may need to be removed from your life ASAP in order to prevent them from doing more damage to you.

Alternatively, especially in cases of semi-intentional gaslighting, it's possible to break free with proper therapy (for both of you, just you, or just the gaslighter) and techniques. However, it can be hard to judge if the person will be able or willing to recognize their problem. Some gaslighters even deny what the therapist says and may refuse to accept they are the problem.

Prepare Yourself for the Worst

Breaking off relations with a gaslighter can be hard, especially in your personal life. If your parents, sibling, or partner are gaslighting you, you need to be prepared to remove yourself from them. The potential hazards of staying are too great, but giving up on a person you love or have become committed to is sometimes crucial. In cases in which total break-off is impossible, reduce the contact drastically. In case you have to have contact with the abuser (e.g., the father of your children), don't let them see that they get to you. Ignore their remarks and act as calm and collected as possible.

Stand Your Ground

Gaslighters need you to be focused on them, and they need to have the power to manipulate you. So, they will do anything to keep you compliant, including making promises that they will stop and/or get help. If you know that they've broken many promises before, don't trust them

Breaking Free from a Work Gaslighter

As mentioned before, HR can be a vital part of solving the issue of workplace gaslighting. As outsiders to the situation, they can gauge what is happening from a neutral standpoint. Asking to change positions, departments, or company locations can all be beneficial to your mental health.

An ideal situation would be to have the gaslighter removed and not you. If it's possible, try to involve more people in the situation. A common complaint may lead to them being removed from the company. In more extreme cases or if you don't have a way to get to HR/someone higher up, you should consider quitting and looking for a new job. Your sanity and mental health are more important than the job.

Breaking Free from a Family Gaslighter

Once again, distance is your friend. You cannot avoid the gaslighter if you live in the same house or even the same city. Family ties are harder to break than work ties. Be careful of potential family gatherings, such as weddings, funerals, and birthdays. If your abuser was in close relation to you (sibling, parent), they might be invited.

In an ideal scenario, your family will recognize the abuse and also sever ties with the gaslighter. In the worst-case scenario, your family will side with the abuser; this will make them gaslighters as well, so you may have to break more family contacts than you anticipated. It will hurt, but you will be better for it in the long run.

Breaking Free from a Gaslighting Partner

Having to break free from someone you love that you've chosen to be with is arguably the hardest of the three. A breakup or divorce is hard to accept and decide on, but those might be your only options. It is not going to be easy, especially if you have been with the gaslighter for a long time. But learn to look beyond any emotional attachment and consider your sanity and mental health first.

Co-parenting with a gaslighter can be really diffi-cult because you obviously can't cut it off with them completely. In this case, you may need to seek professional help to deal with the fact that your partner may get visiting rights.

Stop Seeking for Your Gaslighter's Validation

Most people who are being abused by manipulators will continue to seek the approval and validation of their abuser. Your gaslighter will either give this to you or withhold it, depending on what they want from you. Now that you are working towards breaking free from your gaslighter, you have to silence that yearning for their approval. So long as you are still at their mercy, you will never muster the courage to break free from them.

Breaking free from a gaslighter is not only when you get as far away from them as possible. It is also letting go of your inner desire for their approval and validation. You will also need to discard their views about the world from your mentality. As you stop needing their validation, try replacing it with self-validation and self-approval.

Break Free and Stay Free

When we say break free from the gaslighter, we mean it completely. If it comes down to total removal, you must make sure the break is clean, sincere, and permanent. You should avoid all contact with the abuser; they can still harm you from afar, especially if you let your guard down. Realize that gaslighters are very manipulative people who may sneak up into your life if they find any loophole, and they will stop at nothing to get back in. A gaslighter cannot just let you go like that unless they have found a replacement for you. This is because they are always trying to fill something that is known as a "narcissistic void". This is bad for you because they will make you feel like they want you when in the actual sense, they just want you to fill that narcissistic void.

This is why you need to get away as far as possible and disconnect all ties. Yes, this may mean cutting off contact with a family member, if that's who is doing the gaslighting. It may mean leaving town. But this also means making a sincere and lasting emotional break. You really need to go this extra length because gaslighters can become desperate and hell-bent on bringing you back to them. They can do anything to get you hooked in again, so don't give room for that.

Another mistake that is common with gaslighting victims is trying to maintain contact with their gaslighter. They will just erroneously assume that once they've broken free from the gaslighter, then they can't be harmed by them anymore. Please, for your own good, do not maintain contact with a gaslighter. Most of them have taken time to perfect and master their skills. They will come into your life again, and before you realize it, it will be too late.

Even if they don't come into your life, communicating with them is emotionally battering for you; because every time you talk to them on the phone, see their messages, or come in contact with them, it will bring up all the negative emotions you have stored up for them.

Beware of the Gaslighter's Two-Faced Personality

Once you break free from a gaslighter, it doesn't end there. They will come at you with the appealing personality you knew when you were getting involved with them. That other personality is usually amicable, social, vivacious, and popular, and you can't help but love such a persona. If you allow their charm to work on you a second time, they will tighten their grip when you return so that you will never get the chance of breaking free again.

Also, be ready to not listen to what people around you might say when they hear that you decided to walk out on the gaslighter. I am saying this because the dual nature of gaslighters and other manipulators may get your friends, families, and coworkers to side with them. The gaslighter may present that sweet personality to other people, but it is you who have spent enough time with them that know what they are really made of. If you break free and these people come at you and try to make you change your decision, don't bother explaining to them because they may never understand. They've never seen the vindictive side to the sweet person they know. They will never understand your unhappiness, and they may even take sides with your gaslighter, but do not allow that to bother you.

I believe you've come to understand the instructions I gave earlier in this book on how to find out if the gaslighter is doing what they are doing intentionally or not. If they are doing it intentionally and you have opened up to them that you know what they are doing and they've refused to change, it is time to break free no matter what the people around you say.

Prepare Ahead

One thing that gaslighters do very well is to convince their victims that they cannot do without them, and so it will seem. If you have been abused by a gaslighter, then you know that you cannot just wake up one morning and bail out on them because they've made you dependent on them.

Not just the emotional dependence thing, your gaslighter might also take away the resources you can use to survive when you are alone. They intentionally do this to remove any thought of leaving from your head so they can continue using you to fill their narcissistic void. We've seen women who got caught in a wild romance and married someone only to discover much later that he is a control freak. The guy may have insisted that the woman should be a stay at home mom and take care of the home. If this woman decides that she wants to disconnect from such a gaslighter, she may find it difficult because of the lack of financial resources.

This is why you must plan ahead before breaking free from a gaslighter. If you will need some financial backings when you break free, save towards it. And if you think that you might have an emotional breakdown if you abruptly break free from your gaslighter, then see a therapist that can help you walk through the whole thing and strengthen your resolve to leave.

Practice Peace and Positivity

The times following your separation from a gaslighter might be turbulent for you, so you must have a way of keeping your sanity through the storm. If you are a spiritual person, it is time to draw closer to God and pray more. If you are not, you may need to visit a therapist to help you heal from the damage that the gaslighter might have done. Also, look for ways to engage your mind actively. You can read books, play games, spend more time with friends, and engage in other activities that make you happy. If you are not sure what these activities are, take your time to sample entertainment, activities, and hobbies until you find the one that suits you.

Strengthen Yourself

As you prepare to break free, strengthen yourself. There are plenty of ways you can start growing your inner strength. For instance, if you've not been working or socializing actively, now is the time to do so. You can also try all the wonderful things you have always wanted to try but couldn't because of the abuse you were getting from your gaslighter.

Gaslighters and manipulators generally prefer it when you are dependent on them. So it is very likely that you've been living life on their terms. After breaking free from your gaslighter, try to do everything your gaslighter has restricted you from doing during the abuse. It will help you break free from their whims.

It is very unlikely that a gaslighter will get violent on you for leaving, but if they do, be sure to take pictures and/or record conflicts so you can use them to reveal the gaslighter's true nature and have them pay for any harm they might inflict on you.

Be Brave

The gaslighter might threaten to harm you when you tell them of your intention to break free. Your freedom might not come easily. You might have to fight for it tooth and nail. But through it all, ensure you are brave. If you feel that your life is under threat, report to appropriate authorities and have the gaslighter sign restraining orders.

Also, do not allow the fear of what will happen to you when you are alone to deter you from leaving. Be courageous and believe that you will be fine on your own. It might seem daunting at first, but with the support systems you have built during your planning phase, you will pull through.

Put Your Self-Care First

All of the things we've been discussing so far will not come easy to you, but if you have decided to put your self-care over other things, it will become a lot easier. You can use several self-care practices such as guided imagery, acupuncture and yoga can help you adapt to the changes that you will experience in this phase of your life.

In conclusion, we saw in the last chapter that you can learn how to disarm your gaslighter and still put up with them. But that path requires several therapies, persistence, hard work, and carefulness. So, breaking free is the best option available to you, and you should take it if you can.

Since dysfunctional personality is usually the main cause of gaslighting in a person, you obviously can't change them on your own. Gaslighters wish to control you because they can't control several vital aspects of their own life, so it is only a therapist that can get them to fill those voids in their lives, not you.

TEN

Moving forward - Recovery

A s we saw in the last chapter, breaking free from a gaslighter may be one of the most difficult things you have to do because they have their way of convincing you that you need them to survive. If your mind has accepted this lie, then it becomes truly difficult to survive without them. There is still the issue of getting your sanity and self-image back after it has been bastardized by a gaslighter. You may have a lot on your plate when you break free from a gaslighter, but I will share with you some tips that you can use to recover from gaslighting and regain your normal self.

This chapter will detail the process of healing after getting gaslighted—the recovery, therapy, and moving on with your life.

Seek Professional Help

Depending on the severity of the gaslighting and how long it's been going on, talking to a therapist or a psychiatrist can be a good way of getting back on track. Seek professionals who specialize in psychological abuse victims to get the best treatment.

A therapist will help you get through your emotions. After being gaslighted, you probably have a lot of feelings that you are unsure of and have kept bottled up. So long as these emotions remain bottled up in your mind without you realizing it, you can never be that person you used to be.

A psychiatrist can help you find medication to ease the symptoms of abuse, such as anxiety, insomnia, and depression before you are ready to stand up on your own.

Permit Yourself to Feel

Your feelings were not treated as valid since your gaslighter constantly belittled your feelings and emotions. It doesn't have to be like that anymore. Now that you have broken away from the gaslighter, it is time to learn how to feel again and take your feelings seriously. You don't have to be afraid of feeling anymore.

While allowing your feelings to flow freely, don't

be restrictive. Allow yourself to vent out all the emotions you have bottled up in the past. Don't try to avoid extreme feelings, such as anger, fear, or sadness. It may take a while to get them uncovered, but you must let them pass instead of hiding them. One way to vent off your emotions is to join a support group. In these groups, you can meet other victims of gaslighting and/or other traumatizing experiences. When you hear people talk about their experiences, and you finally start to let yours out, you will surely feel better and realize that you're not alone.

Never Go for Revenge

Sometimes you might be tempted to seek revenge or treat the abuser the way they treated you. I hear people saying you can beat them at their own game. Some people have even come up with steps one can adopt to take revenge on a gaslighter. This is a bad idea, and it is never an option because:

- You will be inviting them back into your life. Now that you have successfully broken free from a gaslighter, the last thing you want to do is to have them back in your life. Don't forget how manipulative they can be. They can gradually work their way back into your life if you're not careful.

- You might be thinking that your guards are intact, and there is no breaking through, but what if I told you that countless victims of gaslighting that I have treated have told stories of how they unknowingly let the gaslighters back into their lives. When it comes to gaslighters, the best way is to disconnect from them completely if you are sure that the gaslighter is unwilling to change, which is very likely. Don't leave anything to chance.

- You will reignite the negative emotions you felt. remember that your number one goal now is to eliminate the negative emotions, not to reignite them. You may feel that getting revenge will make you feel better, but it won't. Rather, it will bring up negative emotions all over again.

- You will give them the option to "prove" that you are crazy. Your gaslighter spent all the time trying to convince you that you overreact and that you are crazy. You knew in your heart that this was not the case. But what do you think it will look like if after breaking free from the gaslighter, you started doing things like trailing a gaslighter and looking for ways to get your pound of flesh? That certainly seems like overacting to me.

- If, in the process of trying to seek revenge, the gaslighter tells you, "You see? I told you that you were crazy," it will hit you differently this time. You might start believing what the gaslighter is saying, and that's returning to the circle of doom. The best thing would be to let the gaslighter be and focus on your recovery instead.

Seek Self-affirmation

Since you've been belittled and your emotions and feelings were downplayed for a long time, take the time to use self-affirmations. It will, in time, help you get back your self-esteem and confidence.

Exercise: start by standing in front of a mirror each day, or by taking a piece of paper if that's more comfortable. Say/write phrases such as "I am loved," "I can be loved," "I am worthy," "I matter." You will probably have to fake it at first, but eventually, you will realize you're telling the truth. This self-affirmation aims to revalidate yourself. It is the most important step in your recovery from gaslighting. When you were being gaslighted, it is possible that you came to mistrust everything you heard, felt, and remembered. You started accepting that you might be crazy. Now that you have accepted that you are fine, it is time to start trusting your instinct and your senses again.

Shift Your Perspective

Acknowledge that you are a victim of abuse, but that you survived it, and you are moving on. Think of yourself in positive ways—as a warrior, a winner, or something else with a positive meaning. What you went through did not break you, and you should be proud of that.

Develop New Relations

You may have issues with trust at first, but you must remember that not everyone is a gaslighter. Try to build new friendships, even new relationships. Take your time and be careful, but not overly so; there are people out there who are willing to help and support you. With that in mind, don't force yourself into anything. Start this process only when you feel ready.

Alternatively, you can start rebuilding the relationships you lost while you were being gaslighted. Recall that the abuser will try to make you turn against everyone that may stand in their way. Your gaslighter will use statements like "So you've listened to that crazy talk that is not good for you, right? They will mislead you soon". Now that you are out of that nasty web, it is time to rebuild all the wonderful relationships you lost during the gaslighting. Reaching out to past friends or family (assuming they weren't the abusers and it won't make it easier for the abuser to get to you) can help you recover and rebuild your life.

Take Your Time

While doing all of the recovery steps we've been discussing, you need to give yourself time. Do not expect to go from a traumatized patient to your former self in a short time. Be patient with yourself and trust your recovery process. Time is the best healing factor when combined with proper professional and self-care.

Emotional abuse is a complex matter. Don't expect to be fully healed within weeks, as it may take years. Do it at your own pace, as long as you're moving forward. Don't try to immediately get back to how things used to be. You must acknowledge that things have changed, and you must develop new ways to deal with them. Don't get frustrated if things aren't moving as fast as you wish they would.

Use Meditation to Enhance Empathy

It is common for gaslighting victims to develop distrust and lack of empathy when they get out of a gaslighting situation. This is because they no longer know who to trust, and, in some cases, they can make them cold. If you have been gaslighted and you now lack empathy towards people around you, it is time to use mindfulness and meditation techniques to prep up your empathy on your back to recovery. I need not tell you that a lack of empathy can ruin the few relationships you might have left. It can also make you act like the very gaslighter you dislike so much, thereby bringing you down to their level.

How then can mindfulness and meditation do this? Let's start our discourse by looking at mindfulness and meditation. Mindfulness is a psychological process that can help you to be conscious of your past and present experiences without judging yourself. Meditation helps you to willfully bring your mind down to the things that matter most to you.

So how can this help you regain your empathy? It works by making you aware that the distrust and cold feelings you have about people in your life is stemming from the gaslighting you suffered. Since mindfulness helps you have a clear picture of everything that is happening in your life, you become aware that your feelings are a result of your gaslighting. Once you have identified the reason why you are the way you are, half of your problem is solved.

The next phase is to use mindfulness and meditation techniques to monitor and track your feelings so that you don't accommodate hates and hard feelings. Since you are meditating and tracking your emotions, you can easily spot those negative emotions and flush them out. To flush them out, you just need to replace them with warm feelings, the kind that is free of negative emotions.

However, redirecting your thoughts will not come easily. It is a skill you will develop gradually using meditation. Meditation helps you to master the all-important skill of redirecting your thoughts easily. The main aim is to remove thoughts that conflict with the feelings you desire. When you successfully flush those ill thoughts, you will achieve inner peace. This inner peace will also show in your relationship with others. When you achieve peace with yourself, you can easily achieve peace with the people around you. Because, now, you are not on edge, and you will not misjudge and misunderstand people's intentions.

Generally, meditation and mindfulness can help you improve your mental health. And trust me, if you have suffered gaslighting, no matter how small, you need to regain your mental health by all means. So, if you wish to become that sweet and thoughtful person you were before you encountered a gaslighter, mindfulness and meditation is your best bet for regaining your mild touch and sweetness.

While there are several forms of meditation, one is more effective for this purpose, and it is known as loving-kindness or compassion meditation. This meditation makes your brain release impulses that breed positive emotions, such as empathy and kindness.

Let's now take a more thorough look on loving-kindness meditation.

What is Loving-Kindness Meditation (LKM)?

Loving-kindness meditation is a type of self-care meditation that can help you boost wellness and reduce stress by helping you increase your ability to accept yourself, forgive others and build better connections with people, amongst other things. We know that before you can't give what you don't have. You must have love within before you can love others. You must forgive and accept yourself completely before you can accept and forgive others. This is the foundation of LKM.

But it can take a whole while to show reason being that the average person is not used to receiving or giving that level of love. So, you may find yourself resisting it, but the key is to keep going until you see results.

Benefits of Loving Kindness Meditation

During loving-kindness meditation, you are focusing and channeling loving and benevolent energy towards yourself and the people around you. Several studies aiming to discover the benefits of LKM have been conducted, and they all yielded positive results.

A 2018 study published in the July/August issue

of the Harvard Review of Psychology gave some scientific insights into the existence of scientific evidence that supports LKM and other compassion-based interventions. In the study, the authors concluded that LKM could be used for treating borderline personality disorder and chronic pain.

Other similar studies have also strongly supported LKM and other meditation techniques as likely treatments for some of the mental health issues such as anxiety, anger, relationship issues.

This is not surprising since another study by Stefan G. Hofmann *et al.* published on Clinical Psychology Review in November 2011 also showed that LKM activates areas of the brain that are directly concerned with empathy and emotional processing. They also concluded that these areas are responsible for reducing negativity and increasing a sense of positivity.

LKM Steps

Follow the following steps to carry out Loving Kindness Meditation.

- Start by finding a quiet place. Sit in a comfortable position, close your eyes, and relax your muscles. Breathe deeply and as you breathe, imagine that you are breathing out negative emotions and breathing in positivity.

- Next, focus on your emotional wellness and inner peace. With your eyes closed, imagine that you are well and fine on the inside. At that moment, try to love yourself and appreciate yourself for everything that you are. Thank you for being a nice person because if you weren't a good person, a gaslighter wouldn't find you suitable for a relationship.
- Choose three to four reassuring phrases that you will tell yourself while meditating. You can tell yourself the messages below, for example:
- "I am sane."
- "I am happy and strong."
- "I am safe and healthy."

You can also create yours, just reassure yourself. Anything that gives you a feeling of self-compassion and warmth is fine. Try to bask in that feeling for a few minutes, and don't allow your attention to drift off to other thoughts. If you catch yourself entertaining other thoughts, gently redirect your mind back to the warm feelings. Do this until you feel enveloped by this thought.

- Imagine receiving love from people that

love you. The gaslighter might have abused you and made you feel worthless, but there are people in your life who have never relented in showing you love. Picture one of them standing beside you and expressing love. Picture them valuing you and wishing you inner peace.

- Once you start feeling completely loved on the inside, it is time to shift your attention to people around you, especially your gaslighter. Extend that warmth and loving-kindness to them. Forgive them of any wrongdoing and wish them good things.

Wish them the best of everything. Let the feelings of kindness resonate within you. Find some examples of affirmations you can say for them while meditating:

- "I wish you happiness."
- "I wish you safety."
- "May you be healthy."
- "May you be strong."
- "May you be peaceful."

Note that it must not be your gaslighter. It can also be people who mean a lot to you, people who have been good to you. It may be your friends, family, or acquaintances. You can start mentioning names and bringing people into your awareness. Wish them success, peace. Reach out to different people you can remember. Reach out to groups of people. The goal is to extend feelings of loving-kindness.

In this case, since you are meditating to recover from the trauma of gaslighting, your focus should be on forgiving the gaslighting and meeting the abuse with loving-kindness. While meditating, reassure yourself that it is not you but the abuser who has a problem. And also realize that they have this problem because of low self-image. Wish them a better self-image and a better heart.

When you are sure that you have removed hate and negativity from your mind, open your eyes. The feelings you just generated should be with you throughout the day. Cast your mind back to it from time to time and try to internalize such a feeling in your subconscious mind.

The procedure described above is just a sample of how you can carry out LKM. It is not an absolute step. You can develop the one that better suits you, so long as it is focused on granting you inner peace and spreading loving kindness.

LKM does not only help you recover faster from gaslighting; it makes you a better person generally. You will feel love yourself more and love people around you more. You will also develop a thick skin against hurt because once you have assured yourself that you deserve inner peace, people's ill actions will not affect you much. Rather you will always meet their unkind deeds with forgiveness.

Conclusively, realize that gaslighting thrives on your uncertainty and mistrust of people. Everything we've been discussing in this chapter is aimed at getting you to be certain about yourself again and to learn how to love again without being gaslighted.

Afterword

Gaslighting is such a heinous crime to the mind of any living human. A gaslighter will make you question everything that you know as being true, which is such a difficult place to be in. If you've been gaslighted before, then you know how traumatizing it can be; but luckily for you, you can overcome it.

In this book, we've taken time to explore everything you need to know about gaslighting. To help you remember the key points, let's go over the chapters again and briefly highlight the important points.

We started with the meaning of gaslighting. We looked at the common attributes of the gaslighter. I said that if anybody makes you doubt your senses or your self-worth in any way, then they are probably gaslighting you. We also looked at the theory behind gaslighting, and we said that a gaslighter seeks control over you because they are areas of their lives where they don't have control over. Fundamentally, gaslighting stems from a bad self-image. We also saw that gaslighting is a type of emotional abuse, one that should not be taken lightly as you can lose yourself in the process of being gaslighted. As a way to give you a complete understanding of the concept of gaslighting, I also shared with you the origin of the word, coming from the play *Gas Light* and becoming popularized through the movie of the same name.

With the basics treated, we shifted to heavier matters. We looked at who the likely suspects are. We identified boss, co-workers, relatives, friends, and partners as likely suspects. I used real-life scenarios to show you how these groups of people can try to gaslight you. My purpose for doing that is to enable you to spot a gaslighting attempt the next time it is thrown your way.

The gaslighters must have a motive for their dastardly acts, what could these motives be? Why do gaslighters gaslight people even when they know that the person might be damaged emotionally in the process of their gaslighting? We identified the quest for total control as the number one motivator for gaslighters. In order to gain control over you, they will plant seeds of self-doubt in you so that you can distrust yourself and rely on them completely. We also looked at the three categories of gaslighting: intentional, semi-intentional, and unintentional gaslighting. We said that unintentional gaslighting is the type that occurs accidentally from a person who is not used to acting that way before. We also said that all of them, even the unintentional gaslighting, is not acceptable.

We went on to look at the symptoms that tell you that you are being gaslighted, and I gave examples. We also identified the common techniques that the gaslighter uses, and they include withholding, countering, blocking and diverting, trivializing, forgetting/denial, and so on. We also identified the common tools that gaslighters use to manipulate their victims. These tools include lying to you, attacking the things you love, discrediting you, shifting blame to you, reframing past events, and using positive reinforcements to calm your nerves while they are on to bigger damages. I then showed you how you could recognize that you are being gaslighted. I said that if you are constantly second-guessing yourself or you have trouble making decisions, if you feel that you are not good enough, if you feel unloved, then it is a sign that you are being gaslighted.

We moved on to look at the changes that your mind can undergo when you are being gaslighted. I said that you might lose your self-esteem and confidence. You may become isolated and experience an emotional shutdown. Then anxiety and PTSD may set in. You become codependent, and you can also develop trust issues and mistrust everybody around you. Depending on the extent of the gaslighting, you may become too submissive or become a puppet in the hands of your gaslighter.

It is not just your mind that experiences changes; the body also does. Typical physical changes that you may experience when you are being gaslighted are insomnia, chronic pain, becoming suicidal, migraines, chest and muscle pains, body dysmorphia, heart diseases, acid reflux, ulcers, and rashes. All of these are results of the anxiety and restlessness that becomes your mainstay.

Now to the key question, "Can you avoid gaslighting?". I said that you could even though it is not as easy as it seems from the surface. We said that the first step to avoiding being gaslighted is getting educated on it just like you are doing now. Then if the gaslighter has started meting out their manipulations on you already and you are not sure of what is going on, I recommended that you get outside advice. I said that you should allow the gaslighter to get you to distrust other people because if they achieve that, you will be at their mercy since there is nobody to validate what you feel. We also said that you could work towards removing yourself from the situation that is causing you to be gaslighted.

We also looked at the ways you can disarm a gaslighter. This is important in cases where you cannot disconnect completely from a gaslighter like when you are co-parenting with them or when you work together with them in a place where you just can't leave like that. I said that in such cases, you can disarm the gaslighter by keeping a log of events so that they won't succeed at getting you to doubt your memory ever again. We also said that you could get somebody to witness your conversations in case the gaslighter tries to distort past conversations. While trying to keep track of conversations with the gaslighter, you must get in touch with your intuition and feelings. You can use active journaling and meditation to get back to your thoughts. I also said that it is important for you to give what is happening a name and avoid confrontation with the gaslighter.

Sometimes, disarming the gaslighter is not enough, especially in cases where you can break free from them. In such a case, I gave you tips that you can use to break free from a gaslighter. We looked at how to do it if the gaslighter is a coworker, relative, or partner. We said that it is not going to come easy, but you must be ready to stand your ground and brace up for the worst. Leaving a gaslighter is not going to be a stroll in the park, but with the right motivation, which is your self-care, you will get out of that abusive relationship.

After breaking free from a gaslighter, what happens next? It is time to recover from it all and get back to your usual self. I said you should seek professional help, give yourself permission to feel again, and never seek revenge. You also need to shift your perspective and develop new relations to help your recovery process. I need to remind you that your recovery will not happen overnight. They say time is the best healer, and it is true in this case. However, you can use the tips we've discussed to hasten the healing.

I hope that you will use the principles you have learned here to break free from any gaslighter in your life.

Do not feel sorry for yourself if you've been a victim of gaslighting. Realize that you are a good person, which is why the gaslighter found you suitable for their manipulation in the first place. But now that you have freed yourself from them, you can go on being a nice person without ever allowing anybody to mistake your kindness for weakness. The world needs good people like you, so keep it up.

One last thing, a favor

Thank you for buying my book. I'm positive that if you just follow what I've written, you will be on your way to overcoming whatever difficulties you're facing right now.

I have a tiny favor to ask. Would you mind taking a minute to write a review on Amazon about this book? I check all my reviews and love to get feedback (that's the real reward for my work—knowing that I'm helping people).

Also, if you have any friends or family who might enjoy this book, spread the love and tell them about this book!

Now, I don't just want to sell you a book—I want to see you use what you've learned to overcome gaslighting and have succeeded in opening a brand-new chapter in your life.

As you work toward your goals, however, you'll

probably have questions or may run into some difficulties. I'd like to be able to help you with these! I
don't charge for the help, of course, and I answer
questions from readers every day.

Here's how we can connect:

Email: June@AtmosPublishing.com

Keep in mind I get a lot of emails every day, and
answer everything personally, so if you can keep yours
as brief as possible, it helps me ensure everyone gets
helped!

Thanks again and I wish you the best!

June

Sources

Aconsciousrethink.com (n.d). *What Gaslighting Looks Like: 22 Examples To Be Watchful Of.* Retrieved from https://www.aconsciousrethink.com/6766/ gaslighting-examples/

Ashworth et al. (2014). *An exploration of compassion focused therapy following acquired brain injury. Psychology and Psychotherapy: Theory, Research, and Practice.* Retrieved from Researchgate: https://www.researchgate.net/ publication/264792392_An_exploration_of_compassion_focused_therapy_following_acquired_brain_injury

Avila, T. (2019). *How Do You Know You're The Victim Of Gaslighting At Work?* Retrieved from GirlBoss: https://www.girlboss.com/work/gaslighting-at-work

Beauchamp, M. (2019). *What Is Gaslighting in Relationships? An Expert Explains* Retrieved from https:// www.mydomaine.com/gaslighting-in-relationships

151

Brocks, E. (2018). *From gaslighting to gammon, 2018's buzzwords reflect our toxic times.* Retrieved from The Guardian: https://www.theguardian.com/commentisfree/2018/nov/18/gaslighting-gammon-year-buzzwords-oxford-dictionaries

Coburn, J. (2018). *Healing From Gaslighting.* Retrieved from https://medium.com/invisible-illness/healing-from-gaslighting-b90dbf23dbaa

Denis, M.J. (2016). *Why People Gaslight.* Retrieved from https://beyondbetrayal.community/why-people-gaslight/

DiGiulio, S. (2018). What is gaslighting? And how do you know if it's happening to you? Retrieved from NBC News https://www.nbcnews.com/better/health/what-gaslighting-how-do-you-know-if-it-s-happening-ncna890866

Duignan, B. (n.d). *What Is Gaslighting?* Retrieved from https://www.britannica.com/story/what-is-gaslighting

GoodTherapy.org (n.d). *Gaslighting.* Retrieved from GoodTherapy https://www.goodtherapy.org/blog/psychpedia/gaslighting

Gordon, S. (2019). *15 Ways to Tell If Someone Is Gaslighting You.* Retrieved from VeryWellFamily: https://www.verywellfamily.com/is-someone-gaslighting-you-4147470

Hartwell-Walker, M. (2018, November 5). *7 Ways to Extinguish Gaslighting.* Retrieved from PsychCentral: https://psychcentral.com/blog/7-ways-to-extinguish-gaslighting/

Healthline.com (n.d). *How to Recognize Gaslighting and Get Help.* Retrieved from https://www.healthline.com/health/gaslighting

Healthline.com (n.d). *What Are the Short- and Long-Term Effects of Emotional Abuse?* Retrieved from https://www.healthline.com/health/mental-health/effects-of-emotional-abuse#short--term-effects

Lambert, C. (2019, April 17). *Gaslighting in Relationships: Seven Ways to Protect Yourself.* Retrieved from PsychologyToday: https://www.psychologytoday.com/us/blog/mind-games/201904/gaslighting-in-relationships-seven-ways-protect-yourself

Lee, R. (2015). *How to Understand Gaslighting.* Retrieved from https://psychcentral.com/blog/how-to-understand-gaslighting/

Leigh, D. (2016, May 20). *How To Prevent, Recognize And Recover From Gaslighting.* Retrieved from iHeartIntelligence: https://iheartintelligence.com/prevent-gaslighting/

Linda, D. (2012). *How to Turn Off the Gaslight Effect in Your Relationship.* Retrieved from EmotionalAffairJourney: https://www.emotionalaffair.org/how-to-turn-off-the-gaslight-effect-in-your-relationship/

Luna, A. (n.d.). *You're Not Going Crazy: 15 Signs You're a Victim of Gaslighting.* Retrieved from LonerWolf: https://lonerwolf.com/gaslighting/

Mcauliffe, K. (2019, February 21). *Gaslighting 101: Are You Being Manipulated at Work?* Retrieved from

Career Contessa: https://www.careercontessa.com/advice/gaslighting-in-the-office/

McQuillan, S. (2019). *Gaslighting: What Is It?* Retrieved from Psycom: https://www.psycom.net/gaslighting-what-is-it/

Neilson, K. (2019). *Gaslighting at work: how do you manage it?* Retrieved from Enterprisecare: https://www.enterprisecare.com.au/newsletter/gaslighting-at-work-how-do-you-manage-it/

Nunymiss, A. (2019, April 23). *One Way to Disarm Gaslighters: Understand DARVO.* Retrieved from Medium: https://medium.com/the-ascent/one-way-to-disarm-gaslighters-understand-darvo-8e0aeb184f7

Sarkis, S. (2018, June 30). *How to Get a Gaslighter to Listen to You.* Retrieved from PsychologyToday: https://www.psychologytoday.com/us/blog/here-there-and-everywhere/201806/how-get-gaslighter-listen-you

Seidman, B. (2019). *The hidden abuse that can hurt your mental health: Gaslighting.* Retrieved from https://www.today.com/health/hidden-abuse-can-hurt-your-mental-health-what-gaslighting-t163927

Sonia. (2012, June 1). *Repair Your Reality After Gaslighting.* Retrieved from TraumaHealed: https://traumahealed.com/articles/repair-your-reality-after-gaslighting/

Stern, R. (2019, January 3). *Robin Stern.* Retrieved from Vox: https://www.vox.com/first-person/2018/

12/19/18140830/gaslighting-relationships-politics-explained

Wanis, P. (2016). *20 Signs That You Are Being Gaslighted – Beware of Gaslighting*. Retrieved from https://www.patrickwanis.com/20-signs-that-you-are-being-gaslighted/

Wilding, M. (2018, June 8). *How to Navigate Gaslighting at Work*. Retrieved from Forge: https://forge.medium.com/how-to-navigate-gaslighting-at-work-bb91ce18ab56

Wikipedia (n.d). *Gaslighting*. Retrieved from Wikipedia: https://en.wikipedia.org/wiki/Gaslighting

Printed in Great Britain
by Amazon

57426746R00102